Throwaway Players

The Concussion Crisis
From Pee Wee Football to the NFL

by
Gay Culverhouse
Former President of the Tampa Bay Buccaneers

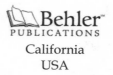

Behler™
PUBLICATIONS
California
USA

Behler Publications
California

Throwaway Players: The Concussion Crisis From Pee Wee Footbaall
to the NFL
A Behler Publications Book

Copyright © 2012 by Gay Culverhouse
Cover design by Cathy Scott – www.mbcdesigns.com
CTE brain scan used with permission from Ann McKee, MD, Boston University Center
for the Study of Traumatic Encephalopathy/ Bedford VA Hospital

Library of Congress Cataloging-in-Publication Data

Culverhouse, Gay.
   Throwaway players : concussion crisis from pee wee football to the NFL / Gay Culverhouse.
      p. cm.
   Summary: "The NFL insists players know they're playing a dangerous game, but players never see the deteriorated
mental capacities of their former heroes.Throwaway Playersis former Tampa Bay Buccaneers president Gay
Culverhouse's story of the broken bodies and lost souls of the men who have left the locker room and what remains
after the cheering subsides. Focused on making money rather than the well-being of their players, this is the dark side
of football the NFL doesn't want fans to see. Additionally, high schools, colleges, and independent sports organizations
have little oversight when choosing player's equipment. This breeds a new generation of kids suffering from multiple
concussions and damaged lives.Throwaway Playersoffers guidance to parents navigating the world of competitive
sports as well as advocacy and resources for athletes often left in the dark about appropriate procedures for treating
injuries, especially head traumas.Throwaway Playersis essential reading for any parent, athlete, and sports fan. Gay
Culverhousetestified before Congress on football head injuries and successfully changed the policy of including an
independent neurologist on the sidelines of every NFL game. Gay's work with former players has appeared inThe New
York Times,Sarasota Herald Tribune,St. Petersburg Times,The Tampa Tribune,Timemagazine, and many more. She
has appeared on several radio shows, including PBS and ESPN, and three documentaries are in post-production (with
CNN, ESPN, and an independent filmmaker). In November 2009, Gay formed The Gay Culverhouse Players' Outreach
Program, Inc., a nonprofit organization to further the work nationally for retired players"-- Provided by publisher.
   ISBN-13: 978-1-933016-70-2 (pbk.)
   ISBN-10: 1-933016-70-1 (paperback)
   1. Football injuries--United States. 2. Brain--Concussion--United States. 3. Sports medicine--United States. 4.
Football--Moral and ethical aspects--United States. I. Title.
   RC1220.F6.C85 2011
   617.1'027--dc23
                        2011017966

FIRST PRINTING

ISBN 13: 978-1-933016-70-2
e-book ISBN 978-1-933016-73-3

Published by Behler Publications, LLC
Lake Forest, California
www.behlerpublications.com

Manufactured in the United States of America

Table of Contents

DEDICATION

Dear Readers,

I write this book in dedication to the members of the Buccaneer teams from 1976 to 1994. You are my extended family and the reason for my passion to change the National Football League.

Your stories allow me to shine the light on the underbelly of America's sport. I do not want to kill the game of football; I only want to make it safer. Violence is endemic to our society, but there are ways to soften the blows. Failing that, we need to care for our gladiators. Right now they are being fed to the lions of bankruptcy, arthritis, and dementia.

I have suffered emotionally in writing this book. I have become angry and frustrated. Testifying before the House Judiciary Committee satisfied me for a moment. I got the opportunity to open the lid on the NFL's treatment of players. However, I shall not be satiated until I can right the wrongs.

Call it guilt. Call it passion. This book was written because of my players, but I owe *all* players.

I want you to walk with me through my learning curve. I want you to see how the puzzle pieces fit together. It's the logical history of a young man's demise at the hands of the National Football League.

I want you to see what I saw — the stark reality that the NFL didn't care about their players once they were no longer on the field.

The players, beginning in high school and college, go to great extremes to become professionals in the NFL, and they damage their bodies with performance enhancing substances in this quest.

In acknowledgement of their willingness to entertain the fans around the world, with or without the knowledge they were sacrificing their future and health, I pledge the proceeds of this book to the Gay Culverhouse Players' Outreach Program (GC POP). My non-profit organization has as its mission:

> The Gay Culverhouse Players' Outreach Program is a non-profit organization, formed to provide information and assistance, at no cost, to former National Football League players and their families, regarding the benefits to which they are entitled.

> The Players' Outreach Program is an outgrowth of the ideas and passionate pleas of its founder, Dr. Gay Culverhouse, to raise awareness and fulfill a need for former professional football players to obtain benefits due to injuries sustained during their playing careers.

> The program will be a resource for former players and their families for years to come.

Our website www.playeroutreachprogram.com will allow former players and/or their supporters to get the information necessary to access NFL benefits. Directions are posted online as well as a toll-free number for personal advice or questions.

Our staff will search for players reported to be homeless or on the streets. Our goal is to serve all players regardless of their mental or physical state. We are an action oriented group.

With your help, we shall succeed. Call our 800 number or visit our website to report a former player in need. If you are a former player, you may be entitled to NFL funds. Check out our website or call.

Please do not think I am resting with this accomplishment. I am going to press for more realistic benefits. No retired player should be homeless; no player should be alone with physical or cognitive disabilities

My next step, as a knowledgeable advocate, is to reduce the number of concussions on the field. I think we are making progress with the NFL on forcing teams to give players a chance to heal from their concussions. Shortly after my testimony, evaluations of competency by neutral neurologists were required to okay players' return to the game. Players who were thought to have suffered a concussion couldn't return to the field that day. The NFL's competition committee recently proposed several new rules that are designed to eliminate head on head tackling and other dangerous plays. They are also discussing less strenuous practices during the week to reduce injuries.

We need to change players' contracts. Players should not have to hide their concussions or injuries to benefit from their contracts. Performance based contracts that are back-end loaded are causing harm. If a player voluntarily takes himself out of a game or self-reports a concussion and is removed from the game, he will not meet his required number of yards gained or tackles or interceptions. This becomes an expensive loss for an incentive based contract.

I shall not stop until I am forced to stop. At that point, my organization will continue what I have begun. I may not live as long as I'd like. I shall, however, rest in the knowledge that I have made a difference in the lives of some.

Most Sincerely,
Gay Culverhouse

Preface

The Day Demetrius (Demo) DuBose Died

PUZZLING END TO LIFE OF INTENSITY
(*The Seattle Times*. 8-8-1999. Glen Nelson)

ROUGHSTUFF:
John Lynch Likes Friend's Life Confrontation, But He Will Never Understand the One That Took His Best Friend's Life
(*Chicago Sun-Times*. 11-19-2000. Alan Grant)

FINAL HOURS OF DUBOSE'S LIFE RECOUNTED--- QUESTIONS LINGER OVER DEATH AFTER CONFRONTATION WITH POLICE
(*The Seattle Times*. 7-30-1999. Alex Fryer)

DUBOSE SHOOTING RULED JUSTIFIED BY SAN DIEGO DISTRICT ATTORNEY
(*The Seattle Times*. 11-01-1999. Alex Fryer)

I read the headlines and cried. Demetrius DuBose was my friend. The Buccaneers drafted him out of Notre Dame in April 1993. He was the fifth player taken in the second round, a linebacker. He graduated from college in three and a half years with a double major in government and international relations. While playing for the fighting Irish, he was one of their captains and an All American. An incredibly well-rounded young collegian, he traveled internationally to Asia, Europe, and South America. He interned on Wall Street. He was planning his post-football career even as he embarked on his professional football journey. He was a man who was going places; he had a real future.

I met Demetrius after the draft. He was attractive, polite, and appreciative of the time I spent to acquaint him with Tampa and his surroundings. He was a gentleman who opened doors for me and asked intelligent questions, along with always being neatly attired and sporting a gorgeous grin. We knew our time together would be short because once he was officially part of the team there would be no time. So we made the most of what little time we had.

We progressed from geographical lessons to fun topics. I taught him about Florida's cattle industry and showed him how to herd cattle. We fished together and rode horses with friends. I even let him drive my Corvette.

Demetrius was special. He reminded me of my son, who was tall and always ready with a smile. But he was more than just a smile. His intelligence shone through, and he could speak on any topic. He was a joy, and best of all, he was eager to get on the field. I was just as eager to see him play.

Once the season began, we waved at each other in the halls, but our times together had come to an end. He was now an employee with a job to do. He became fast friends with John Lynch, another rookie, and they started their careers together on special teams. They were both very physical players and were known to hit hard. Along with hitting hard, they took their hits as well, and they both received their fair amount of concussions during their beginning years with the Bucs.

The following year my father died, and the team was sold. I moved on with my career but often thought of Demetrius and other players with whom I had a special bond.

Demetrius played the average of four years in the National Football League. He played back-up to Hardy Nickerson who was a pro-bowler. Therefore, Demetrius played the suicide position on special teams the majority of his career. He was often injured on

Sunday, was placed on Injured Reserve, and removed by Thursday to compete on Sunday. It was hard on his body. When he left the NFL, he wandered through a number of options but always seemed to have money. But then the unimaginable happened:

On July 24, 1999, DuBose capped off a day of volleyball by drinking a few beers. In the preceding weeks, he had been working out with a trainer, shedding weight and gearing up for his run at the pro circuit. On this afternoon, he had left the beach with a friend who had an apartment nearby. At some point, DuBose crossed the friend's balcony, entered the apartment next door and decided to nap. When the owner of the place returned, he discovered the sleeping stranger and called the police.

DuBose left without argument, and when two police officers arrived, they found him on the street. They tried to handcuff him but he resisted. Then he started to run and the officers pursued him. According to police reports, DuBose then charged the officers with a pair of nunchucks he had wrestled away from them. Eight witnesses contradicted the official findings that DuBose charged the police. Both officers opened fire, and DuBose fell dead. An autopsy recovered twelve bullets, five from his back. The autopsy also determined DuBose had cocaine, ecstasy and alcohol in his bloodstream.

~Alan Grant, *Chicago Sun-Times*

I could not leave this alone. These were not the actions of the man I knew. This was not my Demetrius.

What happened?

To this day, I am haunted. But I think I have figured out what happened to my friend. It has taken me over three years of research; some of it heartbreaking. However, I have intimately lived football, and I am a researcher by training. More to the point, I know the National Football League and I know the practices in the locker room. This skill set allows me to analyze what happened to Demetrius as well as other players who are no longer who they once were. It is quite simple in fact.

Steroids.

Few men are imbued with a natural body of lean muscle mass and the ability to heal injuries in a matter of hours. Steroids afford this opportunity to the ordinary man. Athletic ability is mandatory, but performance enhancers give one the edge.

Aggression, impulsivity and invincibility are the by-products of steroid use. The violence on the field is the result of a physical game enhanced by the warrior mentality steroids promote. Injuries are the result of large men hitting large men. When the hits are to the head, concussions occur. Concussions can lead to Chronic Traumatic Encephalopathy (CTE) which is basically dementia. Demented men do not make good choices. Without intervention they die. This is a logical progression. The unfortunate thing is that it starts at age fourteen with middle school children trying to emulate their favorite players.

I had seen the death of a good man, and I couldn't help but wonder where it began for Demetrius. Had it begun in his early teens? I needed to research more to understand what happened to my friend – and to what is happening to kids throughout the country.

1
Violence On and Off the Field: How It All Starts

My initial research took me to the ultimate original culprit: Violence.

The spilling of blood and the maiming of man have been drawing crowds since before crucifixions were publicly held – and serves as the historic precursor to a growing national crisis. Thieves, criminals and those perceived to be against the ruling powers were hung on wooden structures to die a prolonged death, and the crowds swarmed to these public demonstrations.

Likewise, crowds converged to arenas, coliseums, and stadia to witness Christians being fed to the lions in Rome. Similarly gladiators were fighting for their lives long before the Chicago Bears took the field. The crowds were involved in "the thumbs up or thumbs down" decision as to which gladiator would live to fight again. A festival atmosphere prevailed with the fans cheering for their favorite warriors while being served wine and food. At the end of the day, success was determined by who fought well and who was killed. Violence was the ultimate crowd pleaser, and it continues today in virtually every sport.

And no sport can beat football for excitement. Every few seconds there is a play on the field pitting 300 pound men up against each other in a battle to reach the quarterback and stop the team from scoring. The air is electrified. Fans are dressed in their team logos: Lions, Bears, Panthers, Jaguars,

Bengals, Broncos, Cowboys, Redskins, Texans, Titans, Giants, and they've come to win: "Sack the quarterback! Kill 'em!" The intensity escalates as the game progresses: tackles become stronger, hits become harder. Suddenly there is quiet in the stands. A player is down.

The surgeon who operated on Kevin Everett was quoted as saying Kevin "sustained a 'catastrophic' and life-threatening spinal-cord injury while trying to make a tackle during the Buffalo Bill's season opener, and is unlikely to walk again." The doctor repaired a break between the third and fourth vertebrae and also took some of the pressure off the spinal cord. Everett had a bone graft and the doctors inserted a plate with screws and two small rods to stabilize his spine. Dick Jauron, Everett's coach, discussed the fear that comes from playing a violent game in an article by Dave Goldberg (Associated Press, September 10, 2007). "Having been fortunate enough to play the game and having coached it for a number of years, you don't go into it without knowing that something can happen," said Jauron. "It isn't something they (players) haven't thought about at some time during their careers."

The most famous tackle has to be that of Oakland Raiders' Jack Tatum in an exhibition game at Oakland Coliseum on August 12, 1978. New England Patriot Darryl Stingley was a twenty-six year old star receiver when he collided with Tatum head-on as he and Tatum leapt for a pass. Stingley spent the rest of his life as a quadriplegic in a wheelchair. He died at age fifty-five of complications from his injury.

On November 17, 1991, in a game against the Los Angeles Rams, Mike Utely of the Detroit Lions was paralyzed while playing on the offensive line. When asked in 1992, if he would play football again if he could, he answered, "Most definitely I would. It's what I've done since I was a little rug rat." (Associated Press. "Sports People: Football, No Regrets, Says Utely." January 11, 1992).

On December 21, 1997, the Lions and the Jets were in a battle for the playoffs. It was a powerful day with the fate of both teams on the line. They had worked all season for this day, and the Super Bowl was one game away. Then the game stopped. Reggie Brown, a second year linebacker, fell to the ground. The players scrambled for the team doctors and the trainers. The EMT's were called with their ambulance. Brown lay on the field for twenty minutes. Later at the hospital he responded to treatment for his spinal contusion, but he never took the playing field again. It was too dangerous to complete his career in football.

The most replayed event in football history is the pile-up of the Giants lead by Hall of Famer Lawrence (LT) Taylor on Redskin's quarterback Joe Theismann. Every football historian can tell you it was a home game televised on Monday Night Football. It was an exiting match-up, although no scores had been made in the second quarter. Theismannn, trying a trick play, was overwhelmed by LT. The following pile-up made for one of the most distressing moments in football. As Rick Weinberg of ESPN.com described the scene, "The TV camera zooms in and gets closer and closer and boom—there it is: One of the most hideous sights in sports history. There is Theismann, writhing on the ground, his leg behind him. The bone in his leg is gruesomely visible. Everyone in the stadium and watching on TV turns queasy---or they turn away unable to look at the terrible sight."

Violence on the football field is expected just like accidents at NASCAR races, or blood on the ice in hockey. However, violence off the field is the stuff of headline news. That is not the publicity teams want. It's what teams try to avoid. My goal was to maximize our players' on-field performance status. We called press conferences to announce records set or yards gained or pass/interception percentages. We did not, however, draw attention to the fact that a player beat his girlfriend, or was on the injured reserve list because his wife stabbed him. Wives and girlfriends got beaten. They didn't understand that violence is a part of a player's DNA. How could they?

The man you met in college or at a local bar in the off-season is not the man you live with during football season. The stress to hold his position creates unbearable pressure. The use of performance enhancers change his personality into an aggressive one who stands ready to do battle at a moment's notice. If the player doesn't feel like you understand him, he argues, fights, or leaves. This is also when he finds trouble. There are always people willing to goad a player into a fight. "Hey, how could you miss that pass? Are you blind?" Then there are the new friends who want to drink with the player and bring him down to their level, to get him in fight and then brag about it when the police are called.

There is always the sycophant woman waiting for a lonely player. She calls him "the greatest." He's always been her hero. Within ten months, he's paying child support for the next eighteen years of his life based on his current income.

The pressure on the players is immense. The average time one is an NFL player is four years. Think of all the rookies that never returned for that second year, or who were cut early in their career. It's difficult to recall their names as the press did not have time to follow their career. There was no career. If the average is four years, and some players are on the field for seven to twelve years, think how many players were barely on the turf. Although the salaries seem monumental, consider that a player has, in general, four years or less to make enough money for himself and his family to live on for the rest of their life. In that perspective, it seems a pittance. This is the pressure that leads players to go back into a game knowing they are injured. This is a job. They need a salary.

Rarely do retired players possess college degrees and talents suited to a second career. After a four-year football career, they are still young men, but they are men with aches and pains. They are ill-suited to construction work and physical labor because their bodies have been battered. Sitting at a desk can be excruciating for those players with back problems. These are the physical issues. So not only are they untrained for a second career, they are physically unable to perform most second careers. And worse, money is tight. Four years of salary does not last forever no matter how it is invested. Those players with "names" can promote restaurants or car dealerships, but that doesn't last. There is always a new retired player with bigger name recognition next year.

The league has a week-long program for players who have retired within the last five years, where they learn techniques for securing a job. The NFL recognizes the dilemma facing these young men. One year they are heroes at their university, where they play in a televised bowl game. In April they are drafted in front of a national television audience.

What happens next is anyone's guess.

Player worship, which begins as early as eighth grade, changes a man. He begins to believe he really is as wonderful as his press and his fans think. Ten years later he believes he's above the law and does things wantonly illegal, knowing the laws don't apply to him.

For example, knowing full well that handguns are illegal in New York City, Plaxico Buress, New York Giant at the time, walked into the Latin Quarter nightclub on Thanksgiving weekend in 2008 with a .40 caliber Glock tucked into the waistband of his sweatpants. While being escorted to the VIP section, the weapon discharged hitting Burress' thigh. Within thirty minutes Burress was being treated at New York-Presbyterian Hospital/Weill Cornell Medical Center for the gunshot wound. The Glock was removed from his home, along with other non-registered weapons by police officials. Burress was charged with two felony gun-possession charges. This is simply a blatant disregard for the laws of New York.

Other players such as Ben Roethlisberger begin their life in a new NFL city s a favorite son. Being a first round draft choice in 2004, Ben was humble when he arrived in Pittsburgh from Ohio. He became a fabled citizen by establishing a charitable foundation and donating his time to local groups.

Winning the Super Bowl in 2006 and 2009, the Pittsburgh Steelers came to national focus once again. Ben, as the quarterback, was well recognized and appeared in popular magazines as well as sports pages. Unfortunately, he could no longer fly under his critics' radar.

When Roethlisberger was accused of rape by a woman in Lake Tahoe in 2008, he denied the charges. Actually he went so far as to claim counter-damages.

Continuing to place himself in nefarious situations, Ben was accused a second time of inappropriate sexual behavior. On Friday, March 5, 2010, a twenty-year-old co-ed reported that she had been sexually assaulted by Ben Roethlisberger. This time, the venue was in Georgia where Ben owns a lake house.

Not yet thirty years of age with a $102 million contract, Roethlisberger answered to no one. He demonstrated this in 2006 when he ignored his contract stipulation prohibiting dangerous behavior. Subsequently, he wrecked his motorcycle suffering a concussion as well as a broken jaw.

Roethlisberger's behavior is reminiscent of Kellen Winslow who also defied the parameters of his contract by riding his motorcycle. Learning to ride in a parking lot, he wrecked his new super-charged cycle and damaged his knee. He missed a good deal of the season and had to renegotiate his contract with the Bengals. There was some discussion as to whether or not he would be allowed to return to the team.

National Football League players set examples for college players. The University of Oregon, a Rose Bowl contender in 2009, had a team of players who chose to exhibit their own brand of poor behavior. Borrowing a few pages from the NFL sports pages, and in the period of several months, the Ducks rode the waves of violence both on and off the field.

- During the season opener, Le Garrette Blount punched a player from the opposing team, Bryon Hout, as well as his own teammate, Garrett Embry. He then started fighting with the fans at the game. Coach Chip Kelly suspended Blount.

- On January 24, 2010, Rob Beard assaulted Tavia Jo Ames. A brawl ensued, attracting a crowd. Rob Bear and Mike Bowlin, both Oregon players, were injured in the melee. Beard was knocked unconscious and placed in intensive care at the local hospital. Bowling left the team.

- Acting in a retaliatory manner, Matt Simms defended his teammates' honor and tried to right the situation with more violence. He was charged with misdemeanor assault, and the coach dismissed him from the team.

- On the same day, January 24th, quarterback Jeremiah Masoli and Garrett Embry (dismissed from the team) allegedly stole laptops and other electronics from a fraternity house.

- A few weeks later on February 17, the University of Oregon's top runner, LaMichael James, pled guilty to five misdemeanor charges brought by his girlfriend:
  o 1 count of strangulation
  o 2 counts of assault
  o 2 charges of physical harassment

For the University of Oregon to have this many incidents pre- and post-season, this sends a message to the fans: "Win at All Costs." If a player is disciplined, he must stay in that mode. A suspension is a suspension, regardless of the outcome to the win-loss record.

University of Florida coach, Urban Meyer, held to this principle by suspending his best defensive player for a team infraction. The University of Florida lost the last game of an unbeaten season. Even though Coach Meyer knew that a perfect season was in their grasp, he wouldn't capitulate. Their one loss was the last regular season game as a Gator for many of the players. The Alabama Tide beat them that Saturday, and The University of Florida settled for a win at the Sugar Bowl in New Orleans. The Tide won the National Championship game, capping a perfect season. The players on Urban Meyer's team learned an invaluable lesson. Football does not give you a free pass. No Gator is above the law. This is the lesson we need for all athletes. Athletic talent does not exempt you from decent behavior.

It's expected that broken bodies on a football field are considered collateral damage. The same is true of hockey players, and NASCAR drivers. The participant knowingly takes a risk by entering the field of play. In most physically aggressive sports, the player assumes that at some point in their career, they'll be injured. That's an accepted part of the process. You perform aggressively as there is pressure to keep your position from your back-up on the depth chart.

Carrying the violence off the field is unacceptable. However, it is understandable. For bodies pumped with aggression producing hormones, there is no down time. Their bodies are in warrior mode.

Just as returning soldiers have trouble adjusting to life back at home, football players have that same dilemma. They, like the military men, need support to function off the field of battle. The military provides counseling for returning soldiers. Perhaps the NFL should offer support for players and counsel them how to leave the warrior mentality on the field.

It's psychologically challenging when one is required to be a killer on the battlefield and later be a loving husband. The divorce rate for soldiers returning from Iraq and Afghanistan is higher than that of the average population. These wives suffer the effects of their husband's lifestyles. They are beaten and abused. They are collateral damage. The parallel with the NFL players is striking. Their wives and girlfriends often suffer the same fate as their military sisters.

I don't know the answer to violence. I know that violence on the field is acceptable; violence off the field is not. And yet, we support violence as a way to sustain our love of the game. Is it any wonder that we're willing to look away and ignore what befalls our heroes after the game is over?

2

The Beginning

In 1974, I was drawn into the world of professional football when my father was awarded an expansion team in Florida. However, the true beginning happened several years earlier when, on a Friday afternoon in Los Angeles, my father shook Pete Rozelle's hand. The owner of the Los Angeles Rams had recently died, and my father had a gentlemen's agreement to purchase the team from the estate. The commissioner of the National Football League had confirmed the sale with a handshake. My father was thrilled and envisioned our move to California. That weekend was one of celebration.

On Monday morning my father learned that he had been outfoxed. Robert Irsay of Baltimore was the newly announced owner of the Rams. As the drama unfolded, we learned that Carroll Rosenbloom, the current owner of the Baltimore Colts, funded Irsay in his purchase of the L.A. team. Rosenbloom lived in Los Angeles. Since he wasn't well-liked in Maryland and wanted a team near his home in Hollywood, this was the perfect solution. Within months, Irsay owned the Colts in Baltimore, where he resided, and Rosenbloom had the Rams in California.

My father had nothing.

The glamour of football was over, and my father filed suit against the National Football League. In an out-of-court settlement, my father was to be awarded the next expansion team.

He thought he had won. It was rumored that Florida was slated to be one of the states for another team, which was perfect since we lived in Jacksonville, Florida at that time. It wasn't California, but Dad was satisfied.

Given that he'd planned on buying the Rams, Dad had already consulted financial institutions. Upon hearing he'd be awarded a franchise within the next few years, he solidified the funding to the tune of $16 million dollars.

We waited.

News leaked from the NFL that the owners had chosen two sites: a northwestern site, and a site in Tampa, Florida. Since we already lived in Florida, we assumed Tampa was in our future.

However, given the logic that only the NFL can understand, and being true to their word, the first expansion team was awarded to my father: Seattle, Washington. Further supporting the NFL's logic, they awarded the second franchise in Tampa, Florida to a contractor from Washington, D.C.

Alas, the NFL screwed my father a second time. He turned down the Seattle team, where it was awarded to a well-known Seattle businessman. But as luck would have it, the owner of the Tampa franchise wasn't ready financially. The NFL needed a D.C. presence to lobby Congress on their anti-trust exemption. Their plans backfired when their designated owner could not assume ownership. One had to be prepared to have $16 million dollars in 1974 to buy an NFL expansion franchise (How prices have risen in those intervening years!). Hence, they reached out to my father and offered him the Tampa franchise. Thus the Tampa Bay Buccaneers was born.

Having watched this debacle, I grew to distrust the National Football League. Having seen them make decisions that lacked any form of common sense, I'd become cynical to anything they said or proposed. Back in the 70s they were only interested in themselves. I would always be an outsider, which gave me a unique perspective because I was never in awe of the inner circle that ran the league. I found them to be liars and sneaks.

The lack of respect shown to my father and our family through the intervening years while we waited for an expansion team was quite apparent. Awarding my father the Seattle franchise instead of the team in his backyard was an affront of giant proportions. Who could trust a group that operated in this manner of little respect? We were outsiders, and they wanted to keep us out. If the deal hadn't fallen through for Tampa, my family would still be on the NFL sidelines. Don't think for a moment that my father or I ever forgot that point.

When I attended owners' meetings I was cordial, but I never trusted a word I heard. The deals in the backrooms were driving the league. The rest was for show. It sounds harsh, but I had a front row seat to how our family was the target of this exclusive deal making in trying to keep us on the sidelines of ownership.

Another example of those backroom deals is the awarding of the Super Bowl. For all the community support, time, effort, and money, these decisions are politically motivated. The community organizers like to think they have a part in the decisions, but they don't. I have seen the worst presentations win the votes for the Super Bowl, and it's because the owner could come up with a great backdoor deal and traded chits.

You'll also notice that whenever a new stadium is built or renovated, a Super Bowl will appear there within two years. The Super Bowl in 2011 was played in Dallas, in a venue that was not completed. People had tickets, but the fire department hadn't given the authority for the site to be occupied. The NFL wants you to believe that citizens and committees count in the awarding of plum sites for events. That just is not the case. The owners determine what happens and when it happens. After all, it is their money. They run the league and they pay the league employees' salaries.

In order to have the Super Bowl in Tampa, my father had to promise to vote for a particular city the following year, or he had to discuss pre-season games to be played in other stadiums. Don't get fooled into believing that if your city gets the hotel rooms and puts on a good show, you will, as citizens, get the Bowl. It doesn't happen that way.

My involvement with the Buccaneers wasn't exactly planned. I am a researcher by training and education, specializing in mental retardation and special education. I am a diagnostician, an observer of people. Little did I know how much I would rely on my training.

I was working in the college of medicine in the department of child psychiatry when I broke my back in an accident. My father asked me to join the Buccaneers' staff while I recuperated. I ended up staying ten years until my father died and we sold the team. By that time I had been the president for three years.

I learned a great deal during that time. First I discovered that men hated women being in the role of president of an NFL team, or as a decision maker of any kind. Regardless of the fact that I had an Ivy League doctorate, what could I possibly know about a man's game? How dare I make decisions that any man off the street could do better merely by being a male?

It is difficult going into a family business under the best of circumstances, however, going into a world dominated by men and making decisions that affected them was even more of a challenge. Ironically enough, I believe it was more difficult for them than it was for me. My father gave me a job to do, and I did it. I didn't interact with the players, the coaches, or trainers on a daily basis. I ran a business. The business was football. The planning of the season, the travel, the selling of tickets and skyboxes, the advertising, the community appearances, and charitable donations: this was the business of football.

However, the community of men could not leave me alone. They were jealous. They thought I was incompetent. They ribbed me in the media and didn't accept me at their all-male sports club. A good example of my exclusion was the five memberships the Buccaneers held at a local private golf club. My father suggested I use one of the memberships since I was a corporate officer of the team. I tried to apply and was promptly told that only men could be corporate members.

At this time, I was the president of the Tampa Bay Chamber of Commerce as well, which found me sitting beside these same men in boardrooms and doing business at their financial institutions on a regular basis. And they were going to exclude me? So I did what any self-respecting football president would do; I hired an African American female attorney and sued the club.

After much publicity and gnashing in the press, the club allowed women to be corporate members, but they blackballed me personally. The icing on the cake is that these are the same men who would come to me asking if I could get them Super Bowl tickets—as though I would forget what they'd done. The one thing men hate more than a woman in the locker room is a woman in the front office.

The other thing I learned rather quickly was that what you saw on the field wasn't the whole story. Those three or four hours of play on Sunday afternoon were the tip of the iceberg compared to what went into the game itself. There were practices held at least twice a day in the broiling Florida sun. It wasn't uncommon to see men puking on the sidelines and blood on their jerseys. This was a rough sport. Most people aren't close enough to the field of play to hear the crunching sounds of helmet-to-helmet contact or see the torn skin and the yells of pain as a player goes down on the unforgiving turf.

From the sanitized realm of the skybox, everything is exciting and clean. A drink is sipped, and chips are dipped. However, I'm seeing a different picture, where the doctor and trainers are scrambling to get a player ready for the next series, while he's holding his head trying to figure out what down it is and what position he is playing.

The story of Steve Courson's life epitomizes this fanaticism. I knew this man. I watched his demise. Unfortunately I have watched many such players; and I have seen the aftermath.

3
Steve Courson: Larger than Life

In the winter of 1984, the Tampa Bay Buccaneers did a "Toys for Tots" promotion with the U.S. Marines. On that Sunday all the fans attending the game were asked to bring a gift of a new toy, which would be distributed by the Marines to needy children in the Tampa Bay area.

One of the props used to attract attention to the event was an actual tank. It was parked prominently next to the stadium, and it really drew in the fans as an early crowd pleaser. My twelve year old son literally dragged me over to the tank. I was surprised at how huge the treads were. While I was busy appreciating the machinery, my son pointed out a soldier manning the tank. My eyes scanned upward. Yep, Christopher was correct. There sat a soldier in BDUs with his face painted in camouflage make-up, making the guns on the tank swivel as if searching for an enemy.

By the age of thirty-seven, I had seen a lot of promotions, but I'd never seen quite such a dramatic one. We usually saw well-dressed uniformed men and women with Christmas-themed boxes in which to deposit an appropriate toy.

As I studied the scene, I heard someone in the crowd shout, "That's Steve Courson in that tank!" Yes, that was the Buccaneers' starting offensive guard. Now it made sense, somewhat. He was too large to fit in the tank, but he was having the time of his life entertaining the crowd as he pretended he was a soldier in battle. I wondered if the coaches were looking for him, considering he had a game to play in less than ninety minutes. One thing was certain; Steve was a crowd pleaser on or off the field.

Steve arrived at One Buc Place the summer of 1984 having won two Super Bowl championships with the Pittsburgh Steelers. He was a college All-American coming to Tampa and would make an immediate impact on the offensive line. However, when he arrived the first order of business was arthroscopic surgery on his injured knee. Steve had played seven hard seasons with the Steelers, and his knee showed the concomitant wear and tear.

After a month of rehabilitation, Steve was cleared to play. Feeling he had to catch up with his teammates, Steve decided to enhance his recovery and began a cycle of steroid use. Within three games, Steve was in the starting line-up and played the remainder of the season. Although not an outstanding play maker, he was a consistent force on the line, along with bringing much needed experience to the Buccaneer team.

Within weeks of the season's end, Steve was in Colorado pursuing a new passion: power weightlifting. Using anabolic steroids, he pushed himself with a punishing twice-daily workout and became a self-proclaimed expert on using performance enhancing substances. But that wasn't enough, and he began combining drugs and hormones in his quest for a more powerful body. He felt invincible. His program worked. When he entered the Colorado State Power-lifting Championships in the 275 pound class, he placed second.

Turning his attention to the upcoming 1985 football season, Steve's goal was to weigh 285 pounds and, once again, turned to steroids to aid him in his quest to be the strongest player. His goals were to be able to bench press six hundred pounds, squat about eight hundred fifty, and dead lift a crushing nine hundred pounds. At 6'1," Courson was pushing the envelope on reasonable size and strength expectations.

Steve returned to Tampa for mini-camp in May and went through the drills while working out with the team and new recruits. But something was wrong. As several players later reported, Steve would come in from the field and not be able to catch his breath. He continued to sweat profusely while sitting on the locker room bench without showering or changing. There were more than a few concerned, "Hey, Steve, you okay, man?

The team doctor registered Steve's resting heart rate at one hundred sixty beats per minute and immediately referred him to a cardiologist. The cardiologist discovered Steve had a heart ailment. The size of his body was putting too much strain on his heart. The problem was that his heart didn't distinguish the lean muscle mass of steroid abuse from pure fat, and his heart just could not continue to support Steve's over-sized body. His body mass index (BMI) put him in the obese category. Being able to dead lift nine hundred pounds didn't matter now.

In addition to the heart ailment brought on by Steve's steroid use, he suffered injuries to his knees. Power lifting and working out put tremendous stress on his knees, which aren't meant to support nine hundred pounds. Squats are anathema to healthy knees because tendons and ligaments fray under such circumstances. Strenuous team workouts further pushed Steve to ignore the physiology of his joints. Pushing off with his knees as levers against men trying to reach the quarterback he was protecting took its toll. With only one rest day a week during the season for the body to heal, Steve depended on steroids. One of the touted benefits of Dianbol is its ability to speed recovery. At his age, Steve needed the help.

The problem with Dianbol is that one of the side affects is aggression which, in Steve's case, manifested itself in his warrior mentality. The army soldier in the tank was the personification of Steve's view of himself. He became a warrior against football and his own enemy. He became irrational — another side effect of steroid use.

On one hand, Steve knew he had to quit his reliance on performance enhancing drugs because they were tearing him apart physically and causing him mental distortions. He trusted no one. On the other hand, Steve was addicted to being super-sized. He couldn't be a regular man at this point having lived the 'roid life too long.

Steve knew he had to stop the steroid and drug use but liked the results of being strong and large. He wrestled with the idea that he wasn't really strong, and ergogenic aids were doing the work and lifting the weights. On one hand he felt like a superhero and on the other he felt like a fake.

Driven to act on his impulses, Steve became the first player in the NFL to admit to using steroids to enhance his play. It was at this time that a writer for *Sports Illustrated*, Jill Lieber, interviewed Courson who was quoted extensively in one section of a three part article, "Getting Physical and Chemical."

"Steroids are a different realm of drug from speed or painkillers. They enhance your natural ability. They are a building block. They can take you somewhere. I cannot condone steroid use, but I can morally accept it as an aid." This from a man who lost his career is hard to understand for those of us who are not users. It serves to illustrate the insecurity of an athlete forced to rely on his natural talents.

Prior to his use of performance enhancing substances, Courson weighed between 225-230 pounds. That's a reasonable weight for an athlete slightly over six feet tall. However, in the world of football, it is too small to play offensive guard. As Steve told reporter Jill Lieber, "I think everybody faces the question: Do I want to go on steroids? It happens to everyone at some point in their career at every level. It's like you're cheating when you use drugs, but, then again, everyone else is using drugs too. We'd all be better off if steroids weren't around—everybody would be better off."

Although he left football, Steve could not leave anabolic steroids. He searched for a new career as a professional wrestler. He was a miserable man. For the first time since adolescence, he was without the routine and discipline football provided. He did what he always did to cope, but this time to excess. He drank.

Courson continued power lifting, winning competitions, but not reaching the satisfaction he craved. His steroid abuse was taking a toll on him. Although he was viewed by the public as an aberration for discussing his steroid use with reporters, he was addicted to its effects. The fans preferred to believe the players they worshipped were drug free. Their heroes could not have feet of clay. They had to be naturally super human. Steve was an outcast. His fellow NFL players resented his opening the locker room door on the use of steroids. When he indicted himself, he raised doubts about all players.

This conflict was difficult for Courson to resolve. He finally concluded that steroid use in adults should be sanctioned. However, this isn't what the public wanted. While everyone could see players were growing to outrageous proportions, the fans wanted to believe it was due to the athletes' hard work and diligence. Courson was even more of an outcast for his view of medically supervised performance enhancement.

I followed Steve's career after he left the Buccaneers, which was easy to do because he was a colorful character who said what he thought. One morning arriving at work, there was a group of employees gathered in the hallway having a serious conversation. Steve Courson needed a heart transplant. He had cardiomyopathy.

Shock was the first reaction, but as reality settled us, we remembered three years earlier when Steve had visited the cardiologist in Tampa. It was an omen of things to come. The doctor had warned him to change his lifestyle, to give up his drug combinations, to get his life regulated, to quit the binge drinking. Steve chose not to comply. He wanted to be the invincible soldier atop the indestructible tank rolling into battle time and again.

How much abuse can a body take? Steve pushed those limits starting in college. He was only seventeen years old when he arrived at the University of South Carolina to begin football camp in August. He was thrilled to be delivered from the cold of Gettysburg, Pennsylvania. Steve had been strongly recruited by the Gamecocks and was present when South Carolina defeated Florida State University, a national powerhouse, on a field goal. Steve was sold.

He had stars in his eyes when he thought of playing at Williams Brice Stadium in front of fifty-six thousand of the most loyal and demanding supporters in college football. They wanted their team to win, and demanded the best, even though the university was half the size of Florida State University.

But Steve didn't fully appreciate the pressure of playing ball in Carolina. He suffered dehydration, and at 230 pounds and not yet eighteen years old, he was being flattened by opposing players. In William Johnson's *Sports Illustrated* article, Steve says, "I got banged around by older, stronger kids. I knew at the time I had a lot of work to do. I knew I had to go on drugs. I wasn't going to be out there just to be out there. I had to be the best. I only did steroids the summer before my sophomore year. My body went from 225 to 260 (pounds) in a month and a half."

Courson spoke to his teammates and a coach and was referred to the team physician, who wrote him a prescription for Dianbol, an anabolic steroid. Steve's weight increased from 230 pounds to 260 pounds of lean muscle mass on a program of steroids and weightlifting. Thrilled with his new, stronger body, Steve dominated the field. He became the gladiator the fans came to cheer and never questioned the results of his drug regimen. If a doctor prescribed it, the drug must be safe.

The same held true when Steve was drafted in the fifth round by the Pittsburgh Steelers, the 125th overall pick in the 1977 draft. Steve won two Super Bowl championships playing offensive guard for the Steelers, but it wasn't easy. Chuck Noll was known as one of the masterminds of coaching, and he'd surrounded himself with talented players. Steve had to beat his best because the coaches, teammates, and fans expected a certain level of play. He couldn't disappoint. At 6'1," he wasn't going to grow taller, so the only other option was to get stronger. Courson ramped up his drug regimen and began a program of serious power lifting.

By 1983, Steve's body was beginning to show the ravages of the game. During training camp in '83, he pulled a hamstring muscle during a forty yard sprint. Playing at the amazing weight of 285 pounds, Steve injured his knee in the fifth game of the season. He continued to play through the pain in order to maintain his position and his job with the team. Courson continued to practice but was limping on the field. Finally, pain forced him to abandon practice.

When Noll fined him $100 for not practicing, Steve had enough. "I had gone to war for this man and he was prepared to discard me like an old uniform."

Noll wasn't finished. He publicly took Steve to task in a team meeting by insisting all Steve wanted to do was take steroids and body build. He clearly saw what was happening to Courson, but the problem was Steve couldn't be stopped. He couldn't rely on his own body to play the position of offensive guard since it's one of the most intense positions on the field. Play after play, one is up against an opposing player of the same size or larger. These are the strongest men on any team. Steve wasn't of that caliber, so he had to "super size" himself to compete.

The steroids and power lifting stressed his muscles and tendons, as well as his joints. He was going to break down. Pulling the hamstring muscle was the beginning. When his knee was injured, that was a sign that could not be ignored. Coach Noll knew that Steve's career was on the downhill slide and that he was abusing steroids and drinking to cover his pain. There was nothing Coach Noll could do to help Steve. His activities were keeping him from being a successful player for the Steelers.

The season came to an end, and Courson was traded to Tampa Bay. In Tampa Steve found he had to rely on steroids to maximize the healing of his knee. He also needed them to keep pace with the younger players competing for his position.

In 1991, Steve saw his exposé on steroid use in football hit the bookshelves. He laid bare the facts of his usage just as he had in 1985 for *Sports Illustrated*. However, this time his anger was evident. He felt that he had been blackballed by the NFL and fellow teammates for his open stance on steroid use. Both as an offensive lineman and as a power lifter, Steve had benefited from the effects of performance enhancing drugs. He believed these drugs should be legalized. This stance essentially crippled the NFL's publicity machine that maintained the myth that with hard work and diligent training you, too, could be a superhero on the football field. Fans and sponsors do not want drug-powered heroes.

However, Steve would not quit his crusade. On April 27, 2005, Steve addressed a hearing on steroid usage in professional sports convened by the U.S. House of Representatives. "It is hard to understand the pressure you're under to compete," he said. "This is a competition-driven problem. It's really hard to understand that pressure unless you're out there, having to deal with it. It's a race to be the best. And the NFL, as we know it, is a game where size, speed and aggression are very important." As Courson told Congress, "I looked at it (steroid use) naively. It's like the other strength athletes of my era- a lot of us got into them (steroids) and they worked."

The adverse effects of anabolic steroid use weren't known or fully understood by the coaching staff when Courson entered college at the age of seventeen. He was on the small side; the team doctor had something to help him gain some bulk. Who knew the long-term ramifications in the early to mid 1970s?

However, in 1988 things had definitely changed. A federal and state investigation was launched by South Carolina's Fifth Circuit Solicitor James Anders. A federal grand jury indicted four University of South Carolina coaches for steroid distribution to players on April 19, 1989. The indictments charged that illegal acts occurred from 1984 through 1987. The acts included coaches providing money for the purchasing of steroids for use by athletic personnel, obtaining steroids illegally across state lines, administering steroids to improve athletic performance, and monitoring training programs to enhance steroid use. This campus incident was a strong factor in the passage of the Anabolic Steroids Control Act of 1990.

Stephen Paul Courson was found dead on November 10, 2005,a month after he turned fifty. He was crushed to death by a tree he was attempting to cut down. Steve's wife Cathy had died of suicide earlier and they had no children. His black lab was found by his side.

Later a five thousand word letter was found on Steve's computer. He was still upset that more NFL players were not open about their steroid use. "The league's enormous popularity relies on a myth of its players as drug free heroes. The level of deception and exploitation that the NFL requires to do business still amazes me."

If Steve Courson tried out for the New England Patriots' offensive line today, he'd be considered too small. Every player on that line weighs 300 pounds or more. The Patriots are not unusual in that regard.

4

The Use of Performance Enhancers

"My balls never really regained their size. They're kind of shriveled...sex results in a deep throbbing pain." Additionally, Dan Clark, a former Los Angeles Rams defensive lineman, suffered the ultimate humiliation of having to have breast reduction surgery. However, Clark willingly entered the world of gynecomastia (development of breast tissue in males). Along with the man boobs, small testicles, and infertility, he gained thirty-two pounds of lean mass in ten weeks.

The disappointing fact is that steroids work. If they did not produce results, they would not be used or discussed. Steroids increase endurance, muscle mass and strength five to twenty percent. Athletes have an advantage over non-using competitors; their bodies recover faster after strenuous training and injuries respond more quickly to treatment.

Even non-athletes appreciate the benefit of a buff body of lean muscle. They soon become the envy of their male friends sweating it out in their local gyms. The women flock to their hard bodies. Do not be fooled into thinking I am only talking about adults. This behavior is happening in middle schools and among high school students.

Steroid use by high school football players doubled from 1991 to 2003. These self-reported players represent approximately six percent of the total number of high school students in this study who played football. Unfortunately studies that rely on self-reporting are often flawed. Few players want to admit to steroid use. Additionally, only four percent of the high schools today have drug testing programs for their football teams.

I spoke with several high school coaches who, while denying their players used performance enhancing substances, were convinced players on other teams were using ergogenic aids ("any means of enhancing energy utilization, including energy production, control and efficiency").

One such coach said he felt his team had shown up for a game against a college team. The size differential was obvious. He actually debated canceling the game so as not to have his players injured. His players survived but his respect for the opposing coach plummeted.

Another coach told me he did his own drug testing because the high schools weren't interested in testing for anabolic steroids in his city. When he noticed a player showing signs of ergogenic aids, he immediately asked the parents to come in for a conference. He would not condone or support anything other than natural ability on his team. Instead, he encouraged, even insisted, the parents have a doctor assess their son.

The adverse physical effects of steroid abuse, although known, are often ignored by those that use them. Just as when we indulge in sweets, we rarely take into consideration the resulting inches around our waist. We want what we want when we want it.

Athletes focus on performance. Heart attacks which can occur after the use of a performance enhancing drug are not the focus. Anabolic steroids, specifically, can cause many health issues including elevated blood pressure, harmful changes in cholesterol levels, cardiovascular disease, and sudden cardiac death. When high doses of steroids are used for long periods, liver damage may be severe and lead to liver cancer. Acne and premature baldness are usual in steroid users.

Studies done in the late 1980's indicate that glucose intolerance, insulin resistance, and increased cardio-vascular disease risk profiles, cerebral dangers, musculo-skeletal injuries, prostate cancer, psychosis, and schizophrenic episodes among others accompany steroid use.

According to an article written by Adam Trenton and Glen Currier, "Significant psychiatric symptoms including aggression and violence, mania, and less frequently psychosis and suicide have been associated with steroid abuse. Long term steroid abusers may develop symptoms of dependence and withdrawal on discontinuation of steroids."

As a freshman at Yankton College in South Dakota, Lyle Alzado weighed 195 pounds. He couldn't make the college football team. Alzado understood that an academic scholarship was unrealistic, so he began a regimen of steroid (Dianbol) use and a rigorous weight lifting program. Within a year, he had gained fifty pounds of lean muscle mass. By his junior year, Alzado weighed 280 pounds. Needless to say, he attained his goal of a football scholarship. Actually, he more than exceeded his goal; in 1971, Alzado was drafted by the Denver Broncos.

Shortly before his death in 1992, at the age of forty-two, Super Bowl standout and former Pittsburgh Steeler, Lyle Alzado spoke to a writer at *Sports Illustrated*. "I started taking anabolic steroids in 1969 and never stopped. It was addicting, mentally addicting. Now I'm sick, and I'm scared. Ninety percent of the athletes I know are on the stuff. We're not born to be 300 pounds or jump thirty feet. But all the time I was taking steroids, I knew they were making me play better. I became very violent off the field and on it. I did things only crazy people do. Once a guy sideswiped my car and I beat the hell out of him. Now I look at me. My hair's gone. I wobble when I walk and have to hold onto someone for support, and

I have trouble remembering things. My last wish? That no one ever has to die this way."

The scientific and anecdotal evidence is clear. Anabolic steroids have great potential for harm to the human body and mind. So why, in the face of these facts, do athletes and non-athletes continue to enhance their bodies in such a manner?

Insecurity is certainly one reason. In the non-athlete or amateur athlete, usage of steroids builds a body that is composed of lean muscle mass. The gym rat can impress his friends with muscle mass and a body that reflects the he-man status. Women at the gym and bars are impressed with a physique of heroic proportions. This is the man who will protect them. It's an ego boost to be the envy of your friends and encircled by ladies. The user is no longer one of the pack — he stands out. He is no longer insecure. He can take on the world. He's become "the man."

The realities of cardiovascular problems or infertility aren't on his radar scope. He's enjoying the moment and is in denial about the future side effects. Hopefully, when his testicles begin to shrivel, he'll call a halt to his foolish behavior. But then how do you leave the glamour land of a steroid enhanced body? How do you return to average human size and strength? Can one really return to the former insecurity of being average in the eyes of others?

The same is true of professional athletes. Players establish a certain level of play with ergogenic aids. Fans and teams expect that level to continue. Witness, as examples, the players in baseball: Sammy Sosa, Jose Canesco, Mark McQuire. They reached levels of strength and performance that could only be sustained with performance enhancing substances.

When I was president of the Tampa Bay Buccaneers, I was ignorant of steroid use in our players. I had suspicions, but I never looked for concrete data. I ran the business, and the coaches ran the team. However, some players simply did not look right. My daughter, at age eight, was astute enough to observe that several players looked like the Incredible Hulk. She went on to point out that their necks began at their ears and went straight put to their shoulders. Through the eyes of children the truth is born.

My daughter Susan had a favorite Hulk. He was about 5'10" and played on the offensive line. She sought him out whenever there was a team party or she was on the team plane. At charity fashion shows, he was her modeling partner. He retired before she reached middle school.

A few years later, Susan saw him from a distance and was shocked to see her Hulk was a regular-sized man. She was stunned and asked me what had happened to him. I told her that I believed he'd quit using steroids. Not many months later we read that he had had heart problems- serious heart problems. Susan was devastated. How could a man in his early 30's have conditions associated with men over twice his age?

The postscript to this story is that in late 2008, there was a news lead-in on a local Tampa television station: "Former Buc now a local firefighter." I sat transfixed as the image of the Hulk emerged. His neck was larger than his head and his arms were the size of small trees. I cried.

When you've been a giant among men, it is difficult to be their peer. Your identity becomes dependent on your size and strength even at the risk of your health.

Competition is another reason that athletes of all ages use anabolic steroids. There is actually a known trickle-down effect. In order to play professional football, one must be powerful and quick. National Football League teams draft college players with these attributes. In order to play on competitive college teams, one must be powerful and quick. Hence, high school students strive for these characteristics. As a matter of fact, the goal to play in the NFL begins before middle school in the Pop Warner and pee-wee leagues. The pressure to succeed, to be quick, to be powerful and out-sized permeates the male culture from age seven. Fathers begin taking their sons to football games as early as two (ask me about my grandson). These children are imprinted at an early age into the world of competition.

Parents surely play a role in guiding their children as to what is deemed important. Peer pressure is the other strong determining factor. As we well know, at some points friends have more influence than parents. Good friends share...and there is always a rival.

These dynamics form the structure for drug distribution among middle school athletes. Parents have shown rabid interest in pro and college teams. The child wants approval. In some situations, it's a way out of poverty or a reach for stardom.

Middle school students need to succeed as athletes. The competition is strong with rival schools; some rivalries dating back generations. There is performance pressure. There are supplements to give you the edge. Your best friend got them from his older brother. You take them. You become stronger and faster. Everyone is thrilled with your performance.

Hence, the cycle of ergogenic aids begins. No one tells you about shrunken testicles and man boobs. Would you care anyway? You are on your way to being a professional. Your star is rising, but you've taken the first step toward killing your body.

New players enter the NFL through the draft every April. It's an exciting time for fans and a stressful time for teams.

Scouts have been tracking players since high school. They've charted their weights, their speeds, their ability to jump, and their intellect, among other factors. There are doctors' reports to be reviewed and discussions of arrest records. Weak spots on the team are analyzed, and a plan for draft day is adopted. This plan includes player trades and changes in the depth chart.

There is stress in the ranks of the current team members. Who are the rookies going to be? Are they out for my job? Everyone is out for my job. That's what depth charts are: the chart delineates who is in line for your position. If you are injured in a game, you go back in. Why? Because you don't want your back-up to have the opportunity to show he can play the position better than you.

Gene Upshaw, the former players' union executive director, speaking May 9, 1989, before Congress in a hearing presided over by Senator Joe Biden made the following remarks: "I first must say that it is virtually unanimous why steroid use is pervasive it sports...it has to do with pressure. There is the pressure to earn money; there is the pressure to keep a job; there is the pressure to keep ahead of competition; and there is pressure to win."

I spoke with two linebackers and an offensive lineman recently. Their words were identical, "Gay, after the third play of every game, I saw ten men in front of me instead of one. I had to ask my teammate to show me where to block or move. After the huddle, I walked the wrong way. I kept hitting the side of my helmet thinking it would clear my head. Leave the game? Tell the coach? NO WAY! I need this job!"

"Yeah, I've played with broken bones; I taped them up and went back in." Relief of pain leads to another dimension of performance enhancement: Vicodin, Percocet, Dilaudid, etc. If a player, through drugs, can ignore pain then he can play competitively. The coach needs the player on the field. The player needs to keep his job.

Enter the team physician.

There exists in the NFL a lively debate on the role of the doctor on a team. Does he protect the interests of the player, or the team's interest? I have a simple answer. Who pays his salary? According to the NFL, the role of the physician is to safeguard the welfare of the players on the team. However, in reality, this is a difficult stance to maintain.

Speaking recently with a former team doctor, he brought up a point that I had never considered. Being a team doctor adds prestige to your credentials and attracts more patients to your private practice. Only the other day a friend proudly announced to me that he had secured an appointment with the Boston Red Sox orthopedist. In his mind it was a coup. This doctor was preordained to be "the best" because a team had deemed him to be.

What my friend failed to realize was that in these economic times, doctors will work for free to be associated with a professional team. The additional exposure on the field and on television, the listing in the media guide, and the photo in the Game Day program brings revenue to the physician.

Hospitals are known for paying their way into a team alliance. Billboards and advertising, suites, and reduced medical rates are traded for the ability to be the official hospital of a team. Interestingly, the official team physician may not even have medical privileges at that hospital.

But what makes life really interesting is that coaches have been known to override physicians' orders. It's my belief that physicians should be liable for allowing this to happen and thereby sending them back into play.

One such incident was documented by Alan Schwarz in his article for the New York Times (2-2-07) "Dark Days Follow

Hard-Hitting Career in the NFL." Ted Johnson spent ten years in the National Football League as the New England Patriots' middle linebacker. He helped the team win three Super Bowls before retiring in 2005. In the article, he told Schwarz that he knew there was something wrong with his brain. Furthermore, he knew when it started. During a pre-season game in August of 2002, Johnson sustained a concussion. The team doctor and the trainer, Jim Whalen, recommended rest and no contact drills for several days. Bill Billichick, the head coach, went against those recommendations four days later and ordered Johnson onto the practice field to test his recuperation, where Johnson sustained another concussion.

Johnson, his doctor, and his trainer knew it was a bad idea to risk his brain to a second concussion so soon after the first in August. Johnson was trying to follow the orders of the team doctor and trainer. However, Johnson needed his job, and he was under pressure to perform and secure his position for the 2002 season.

Likewise, the trainer wanted and needed his job. Coach Billichick knowingly risked the career of Ted Johnson through intimidation. Who is liable for this injury that ultimately led to the end of his of Johnson's football career and his income? Today Ted is very vocal about the way in which he was treated, and counsels players to take care of themselves. He lives minimally and is in constant pain with searing headaches and aching joints.

In contrast, some players, against medical judgment, beg doctors to "keep me in the game." Coaches, as well, will demand that team doctors get the players back on the field. The masking of pain starts early, according to Jason Peters in his book *Hero of the Underground*. During his freshman football year at the University of Nebraska, Peters was given six Lorcets (also known as Vicodin, a habit forming narcotic and analgesic) by the team doctor to control minor knee pain.

Unfortunately, this is not an uncommon practice. Society itself has become accustomed to feeling no pain. We solicit pain killers regularly to deal with the usual aches that bodies experience. Pharmaceutical advertising takes up a disproportionate share of space in magazines and television. We are convinced that we should not suffer one minute when there is a pill to ward off any unpleasantness.

Football takes this concept to a dangerous level. Pain is nature's way of telling us that our body is suffering. It's a signal to reassess what we are doing and change our behavior to alleviate the pain. Pain keeps us from harming our body, if we listen.

Randy Grimes, former Buccaneer center (1983-92), is a friend of mine. He fights his addiction to painkillers every day. He puts on his good old boy Texan persona and greets each day with a will to succeed; he will not succumb to those pills today. It's not an easy fight.

Randy's drug use started in the locker room. Everyone knew the combination to the opiate safe, and all the players had bowls of anti-inflammatory pills at their fingertips. As a center, Randy was beaten up both during practices and on Sundays. One day of rest wasn't enough time to heal his knees, neck, and shoulders. More and more, he relied on painkillers to keep him on the field and secure his position. He had a wife and children to support. He needed this job.

In 1992, at the age of thirty-two, Randy retired due to injuries and returned to Texas. He secured a job as a salesman for a brick company. However, his drug dependency continued. Randy found the drugs his body craved through storefront medical shams. For $100 he got the prescription he needed. What started as a drug to relieve pain became an addiction. The older he became, the more his arthritic joint pain intensified, and the more his addiction took over his life.

He lost his job for non-performance because his drug abuse was obvious to his bosses. His wife and children suffered as the man they loved turned into a man they no longer knew.

Randy was in a downward spiral as he spent his money to satisfy his drug addiction. He lost his home, and he lost control of his life.

Recently Randy completed a drug rehab program and had surgery to replace his knee. He is hopeful that he can cope with his neck and shoulder pain without resorting to painkillers. He has a workout regimen and is in great physical shape. He is positive about his chance for success. He is hopeful he can mend his relationship with his wife and children.

On a personal level, I love Randy's smile, his teasing, and his light-hearted and fun-filled jokes. He is truly a joy to be around these days. He is no longer angry and depressed. Randy has now become an integral part of the Gay Culverhouse Players' Outreach Program helping us locate players that need our services.

Randy and I email several times a week, but if I don't hear from him, I worry that I've lost him again to the world of drug addiction: a world that started in my locker room. It never goes away for the afflicted or those who care about them.

Pain keeps us from harming our body. When we mask pain, we cause further injury. Unfortunately, I witnessed this first hand. Wally Chambers was at the end of his career when the Buccaneers obtained him from the Chicago Bears. Chambers was tall and lean and possessed a leadership style that the team needed. We also needed him badly to fill a gap in the team. The coaches knew Chambers had knee problems. The doctor said he could handle it. This was an interesting assertion, considering he wasn't an orthopedist. The Tampa Buccaneers were the only NFL team to have a general surgeon as a team doctor. You might wonder how this happened. I do, too. All I can say is that he played golf, as did coach McKay and Hugh Culverhouse, the owner.

Chambers was an immediate starter for the team. Due to his height, he was easy to follow on the field. He knew what he was doing and had a steady presence. However, as the game progressed I could see that he was struggling and losing quickness. During a timeout the team doctor formed a huddle on the sideline with Chambers in the middle. With the players forming a visual wall, the doctor injected Chambers' knees. He returned to the field and made his plays pain free, but at what expense to his health? Was the doctor treating the patient for the patient's good or the good of the doctor's employer?

I recently had the opportunity to speak informally with several retired players, now in their fifties. We were discussing joint replacement surgeries. The players were concerned that the team doctors had given them cortisone injections in their shoulders, hips, knees, and ankles before a game. Additional doses were administered during half time. In retrospect, they were convinced that these medications, while masking pain, had contributed to the destruction of their joints.

I understand the need for cortisone injections. I willingly used them to block the pain of a deteriorating knee so I could compete in horse shows. After two years, I acquiesced and had the knee replaced. However, in my case, I *asked* for the injections. I was told the risk involved and made an informed decision. The former players didn't have this conversation with their team doctors. There was no choice. The results: crippling arthritis.

Congress recognized this dilemma in a one hundred forty-four page report from the non-partisan Congressional Research Service (CRS) recommending legislation to address the health problems faced by professional football players. The report, which was released on April 9, 2008, stated, "…the NFL and the NFLP.A. need to make serious efforts…to eliminate the conflict of interest by team doctors who place the financial interests of their teams ahead of players' health." The report also notes that, "The current system is subject to a variety of conflicts of interest which appear detrimental to players. Medical care provided by the team for its players raises serious conflicts of interest concerns as a team physician must balance the players' health concerns with those of the coaches and owners who expect players to play injured."

On October 28, 2009, I addressed the House Judiciary Committee hearing "Legal Issues Relating to Football Related Injuries" chaired by Congressman John Conyers. The following are exerts from my written testimony:

> From the beginning let there be no mistake, football consists of a series of games being played to determine the ultimate Super Bowl champion. Contrary to popular opinion, this is no longer a rich man's hobby. In reality this is a cutthroat business. The goal is for the franchise to make money. The product is games on the field. The "win" is a positive bottom line.
>
> From this vantage point, the most important insight I can give this committee concerns the medical care of the players. This care is entrusted to the team physician; a man who is hired by the coach and paid by the front office. The doctor has the ability to choose his assistants without interference from the administration.

The doctor reports to the coach. He attends the combine prior to draft day and gives his input as to the status of players' previous college injuries. He is part of the physical examinations and pours over the medical records of the NFL hopefuls. Clearly he is helping the coaches choose the incoming team.

The team doctor is invested in the performance of these players who make the team. He does not want to be seen as lacking in assisting the coach in his selection. The team doctor wants these players to succeed in helping the team win games. The team doctor gets to the point where he will do anything to enhance the performance of these rookies. With very few draft choices, the decisions on whom to draft are critical to a team's success. Hence, from the beginning, the team doctor is invested in the success of their choices.

This alignment is the crux of the problem for the players on the team. The doctor is not their medical advocate. He's not even conflicted. He knows who pays his salary; he plays golf with the coach and the owner, not the players. He is management; he makes decisions for the management side of operations. He understands the bottom line is business. The team that wins sells more luxury seats, skyboxes and fills the stadium. Therefore, more parking is sold on game day along with more beer, sodas and cotton candy. This is the term of success.

If a player suffers an injury, the team doctor's role is to find a way to have that man back on the field the following game, if not the same game. The player is shot with cortisone during the game to see if the pain can be numbed if it is a joint or other such problem....

We have been reared in America to trust doctors....We knew the doctor was on our side even when he told us things we did not wish to hear. He had our wellbeing as his primary mission. Young men in college and entering the NFL believe that the doctor is there for them as well. Why would the rules have changed? It takes the players a while to get the message that they are being asked to play in some situations that are not comfortable. After all, they are viewed as a business commodity not an employee. Then they are being shot to mask pain. At this point they realize the doctor is working for the management.

When a player goes outside the system for a consultation, he is immediately suspect. He is not a "team player"; he has shown that he does not trust the medical staff. He becomes a pariah because he has broken with the team system. Other players who may refuse to practice or play are called lazy or injury prone. If a player sets out to protect himself, he is probably on his way to another team.

In their efforts to optimize players' natural talents, the trainers and team doctors introduced a variety of performance enhancing substances to the team. The doctors and trainers were in conflict with the health of their players. For whom were they working? Steroids were introduced into the San Diego Chargers in 1963 by strength coach Alvin Roy who had worked with the United States Olympic weight lifters.

Matt Chaney's book, *Spiral of Denial*, mentions how in 1935, Dr. Charles D. Kockakian isolated testosterone in an experiment at the University of Rochester. As he studied the testosterone, he realized its anabolic or tissue building nature. Within several years, steroids were used in athletics, primarily bodybuilding and weightlifting.

In 1954, the USSR weightlifters dominated the World Games. East Germany became one of the first countries to use doping as a regular part of the training routine for its promising athletes.

Prior to the middle 1960's, football players were considered quicker and more agile if they were not encumbered by muscle bulk. Alvin Roy changed this theory using Dianbol produced by CIBA and developed in conjunction with American Olympic physician John Zigler. The teams he counseled grew in size and quickness. They dominated opposing teams. Soon every NFL franchise wanted in on the secret.

The secret that everyone wanted was not an illegal substance. It was viewed as a nutritional supplement—a vitamin with special powers. Relative to society in the 60s, it was just part of a cultural trend of taking pills to sleep, lose weight, be happy, relaxed, or remain awake. We were a pill popping group looking to enhance our lives.

Steroids were considered so benign that in 1965, Dr. H. Kay Dooley organized a study involving three commercial brands of anabolic steroids for high school football teams. "If I knew of something which may improve performance…a drug that is legal and which I don't believe involves serious health risks, I see no reason not to make it available to an athlete."

In 1965, I entered university. As most freshmen do, I clamored for the excitement of Saturday's football games. The consuming talk all week focused on the pre-parties, the post-parties, and the total thrill of the day. We were considered a football powerhouse. I say "we" because football was "we." That was our identity. We were on national television, we were invited to bowl games, and we had a Heisman contender. Our coach made more money than the university president.

In retrospect, I realize that we dominated due to size, strength, and quickness. Even the red-shirt freshmen stood out on campus. They arrived from prep play in that condition. They were strong in high school. They were using the supplements CIBA manufactured. And nothing was illegal. Nothing was frowned upon. These men were our heroes. They were literally the Big Men on Campus. It was the 60s, and everyone was happy.

Looking back twenty years, Dr. John Zigler was quoted as saying, "I wish to God now I had never done it (create Dianbol). Steroids were such a big secret at first, and that added to the hunger of the lifters and football players to get hold of them."

Players trust their team doctors and trainers to safeguard them. Isn't it ironic that these are the very men who introduced steroids into the National Football League? Heart attacks and liver cancer, shrunken testicles and infertility are the physicians' gifts to the teams and their athletes.

5
Six Players Dead

Players using ergonomic aids grow to absurd proportions. It was obvious that normal men did not reach those sizes through good diets and routines of exercise and hard work. What was going on in my locker room?

When Steve Courson admitted to using steroids, he was ostracized by teammates who were doing the same thing. This double standard angered him. However, it answered my questions.

Anabolic steroids have the added side effect of making the user aggressive and impulsive. This is a bad combination. Picture a man who is worshipped for his athleticism and his size to compete in the NFL. Fans come up to him in bars and want to buy him a drink or talk football; women want to be photographed with him. Now, add the components of aggression and impulsivity. The aggression serves him well on the field. However, off the field it is a time bomb. Without the ability to monitor his behavior and control his impulses, trouble looms everywhere he goes.

I learned this well. Within a week of being signed, our first round draft choice was caught in a police sting soliciting oral sex for fifty dollars. The players teased him. They informed him that Buccaneers get sex for free. They demand it.

The third round draft choice that year missed several games. His wife was tired of being beaten; she stabbed him with an ice pick.

Our star quarterback was well known at Hooters. He routinely lost all sense of responsibility. The servers hid from him. At closing time, more than once I was called to take him home because he was barking like a dog and crawling on the floor chasing the girls.

Sexual harassment was commonplace. It got to the point where I restricted certain areas in our own offices because I didn't want my staff put in awkward positions. The players had no self-control. They were kings everywhere they went.

Unrestricted behavior enhanced by the side effects of steroids and NFL status lead these men to believe they are invincible. Fights are common, and guns are carried.

Violence is another side effect of steroid use and other performance enhancing substances. Combine violence with size, aggression, and the lack of impulse control, and you have a toxic cocktail that always results in disaster.

There is no better example of this than Adam "Pacman" Jones, whose penchant for violence ruined his career. Pacman is the epitome of the modern, self-absorbed player, but he's not the only player who attracts and causes violence. He is merely an example of what owners and coaches face in their chemically enhanced players.

I can't drive this point home enough; when seeking stronger and faster players, there is a downside. Players hurt one another during the game and damage their careers off the field.

And sometimes, they die.

When Tom McHale arrived as a free agent for the Buccaneers, my daughter was fourteen years old. When he departed for the Eagles, she was eighteen. As any parent knows, these are treacherous years for a teenager. My daughter was adorable, blond, blue-eyed, perky, and friendly beyond belief. It was as though she was constantly and unconsciously running for "Miss Congeniality."

As a mother, I didn't look at her as an object of men's sexual desire. Boy, was I wrong! I was still car-pooling her to soccer games. When she got a car, it was for my convenience since she never asked for one. I thought she and her girlfriends looked cute and wholesome driving to the beach in her convertible. That was my vision.

It was not, however, the vision of several new recruits to the team. Our home phone would ring constantly with deep male voices asking for "Susan." By the hours of the calls, ten p.m. or later, I quickly knew these were not just mature sounding high school friends. I told the anonymous voices that my daughter was asleep.

Magically, within two weeks each season, the calls would cease. I didn't quite understand why, but all was quiet until the following year.

The penny finally dropped when my assistant told me what was happening. (Assistants always know more than their bosses.) Tom McHale would hear locker room talk about my daughter. He'd gather a few other offensive linemen and they'd find the late night callers and school them. "If you want a position on this team, Rookie, you do not mess with the owner's granddaughter." Unbeknownst to me, Tom led the enforcers; he and his line were my daughter's protectors year after year. They ensured her innocence and provided her the teenage years every child deserves. She was free of the sexual pressures of twenty-two-year-old football players.

I wish I could reach out to Tom and tell him what a difference he made in our lives. I was an over-worked, naïve mother, and Tom had my back. He made a difference to my family—a substantial contribution to the well-being of my daughter and to our future as a family.

Why didn't I get the chance to tell him before he died? How could he have died at the age of forty-five? If I had known he was in trouble on May 25th, 2008, I would have gone to him. I would have found help. I would have tried everything to save him.

In a *Science Daily* article published January 27, 2009, I read that "nine-year veteran, former Tampa Bay Buccaneer Tom McHale was suffering from chronic traumatic encephalopathy (CTE), a degenerative brain disease caused by head trauma."

I could not have saved Tom.

At the time of his death, McHale was being treated as an outpatient at a drug rehabilitation center. The official cause of death was listed as an accidental drug overdose after a long battle with addiction. He was self-medicating to alleviate the symptoms of CTE that he was experiencing: memory loss, uncontrollable emotions, impulsivity, and depression. How does one escape the effects of brain trauma? It is impossible. Tom was not getting better; his symptoms were not going to abate. He was heading toward dementia, and there was no return. Expert consensus is that drug abuse of any kind would never cause the neuropathological findings of CTE found in McHale.

Tom McHale graduated from the Cornell School of Hotel Administration in 1987. His first two college years he attended the University of Maryland and played defensive tackle on two Bowl teams. While playing for Cornell as a defensive end, he was named All-Ivy League and first team All-American in 1986, and was runner-up for Ivy League Player of the Year—a distinction not normally accorded a defensive lineman. In 1993, McHale was named to the Cornell Athletic Hall of Fame for setting school records such as career quarterback sacks.

McHale returned to the Tampa Bay area after playing two years with the Philadelphia Eagles and one year with the

Miami Dolphins. Using the culinary and administrative skills he studied at Cornell, he opened two popular restaurants in 1999, McHale's Sports Pub and McHale's Chop House. Tom grew up cooking and barbequing for his family in Maryland. His restaurants quickly became known for helping local charities with fund-raising events. Tom McHale remained the guy with the ready, open smile willing to help anyone or any organization. He was truly one of the good guys.

But under that public smile, his brain was deteriorating. Chronic traumatic encephalopathy can take ten to twenty years to destroy a brain. Playing first on the defensive line and then switching sides to protect his quarterback, Tom took a lot of hits in his nine year NFL career. He became a college All-American for leveling opposing quarterbacks for four years.

Although Tom never experienced a documented concussion, it is estimated that he suffered the equivalent of twenty thousand whiplashes. His body accelerated on the line and then came to a quick stop. His brain crashed against the front of his skull, and then, according to the laws of physics, (for every action there is an equal and opposite reaction) his brain recoiled in the opposite direction hitting the back of his skull. It's the same action that happens in "shaken baby syndrome." Tom's brain was jolted and slammed against his skull so much that his body started releasing a toxic protein (Tau) throughout his brain. This abnormal protein killed his brain cells. Of course, he turned to drugs and tried to rid himself of the dementia that was invading his brain. He didn't know what was happening, and no one could help him.

Tom McHale is the most recent NFL player to be diagnosed with CTE upon his autopsy. In death, he joins a group of elite athletes who have suffered the consequences of repeated brain trauma on the football field.

In 2002, Michael Lewis "Iron Mike" Webster died at the age of fifty. With his death, he became the first player to be diagnosed upon autopsy with gridiron dementia, later known as chronic traumatic encephalopathy. A tragic ending for one so smart.

Mike attended the University of Wisconsin on a football scholarship and maintained standing on the academic honor roll. During those years, he was considered a "most valuable player" and was named center for the All Big Ten team.

In 1974, the Pittsburgh Steelers took Webster in the fifth round. At 6'2" and 225 pounds, he was considered small by NFL standards, and Mike knew he had to do something to change that dynamic. He began a strenuous workout program aided by anabolic steroids.

Within two years, Mike was 260 pounds and the starting center for the Steelers. Within the league, he gained the moniker "Iron Mike" and was universally considered the strongest man in the National Football League.

A six time All-Pro player and nine times Pro Bowl selection, Webster won four Super Bowl rings during his tenure with the Steelers. In 1999, *The Sporting News* named him 75th out of the 100 greatest football players. In 2000, he was center for the All-Time NFL Team. In six straight seasons, he never missed a snap.

Although not specifically treated for concussions during this time, his doctors have estimated that he suffered the equivalent of twenty five thousand automobile crashes during his high school, college and professional playing days.

When he left football in 1990, Mike held eight jobs in four years. He entered several business ventures, all of which failed. By 1996, Mike was broke. This was not a case of "not being able to make it in the outside world." Many former fans like to use this excuse, but it deflects attention from the true problem: Mike Webster's brain was severely damaged.

Mike was an honor student in college. By the time he left the National Football League, he suffered depression, paranoid delusions, extreme physical pain from torn ligaments, herniated discs, as well as arthritis. He became violent and agitated. The loss of his reasoning and cognitive abilities sent him into debt and left him living in his truck. He no longer possessed the ability to make sound financial decisions. He began to self-medicate to alleviate his confusion, depression, and physical pain. His low point arrived in September of 1999, when he was placed on probation for forging prescriptions.

During his 1997 acceptance speech for his induction into the Pro Football Hall of Fame, Webster's cognitive disabilities became apparent when he rambled through his twenty minute speech. His thoughts didn't flow consecutively. The crowd grew restless and then alarmed. It was obvious that Iron Mike was in trouble.

Webster's doctors were convinced the concussions during his career damaged his frontal lobe, causing cognitive dysfunction. According to one doctor, Webster's injuries were similar to a boxer's, and that he was essentially "punch drunk," and that affected his attention span, concentration, and focus, leading him to act erratically. What was worse is that doctors claimed the condition was irreversible, and an operation wouldn't improve his brain functions.

When he died, Mike was living with his son, Garrett, a high school senior who was a lineman on his high school football team.

Justin Strzelczyk met his childhood friend Jim Dolan, M.D., September 29, 2004, at 6:30 p.m. In Leonard Shapiro's *Washington Post* article, Dolan recalls that night, "He looked good. His weight was down, but once he started talking, my heart just sank. I realized he was manic, almost acute psychotic. He was telling me he couldn't sleep, he was hearing voices." Strzelczyk told him he believed devils had been knocking at his door, that the end of the world was coming and that the government was trying to control his life. He thought recent natural disasters were omens of doom.

At eight-fifteen the next morning Justin was killed in a fiery head-on collision with a tanker truck after a forty mile chase on the New York Thruway. Troopers said he attempted to elude police and eventually crashed his pick-up truck into the tanker after driving erratically at high speed.

Donal Faugham was the state police captain who supervised the crash investigation and spoke with Alan Schwarz in his *NY Times* article. "It appears he was suffering from some kind of mental psychosis." Three years later that statement was proven to be correct. Working with brain tissue saved from Justin's autopsy, Dr. Bennet Omahu of the University of Pittsburgh School of Medicine, found "irreversible brain damage...most likely caused by concussions sustained on the football field."

Justin Strzelczyk was drafted by the Steelers in the 11th round of the 1990 draft. In eight seasons he missed only two games, both of which were in 1997. In 1998, he suffered a quadriceps injury. That kept him on injured reserve through 1999. He then left football.

Strzelczyk was known as a player who could fill any position on the offensive line. His play was vital in taking the Steelers to six playoff seasons. Playing long and hard, Justin sustained concussions that went untreated. As 11th round choice, he'd had to fight for his position, and he wanted to play. Players in the huddle with Strzelczyk remembered his vomiting before breaking for the next play. He suffered to play. How many concussions did Justin sustain? Enough so that at the age of thirty-six, he was depressed, delusional, and paranoid.

And dead.

Downing a combination of prescription drugs and rat poison in an attempt to kill one's self seems a particularly desperate action. That is exactly the response Terry "T-Bone" Long had when he was suspended in 1991 by the NFL for violating the league's steroid policy.

During training camp in July, his testosterone level was tested at three times the NFL limit. He was suspended for four games once the season began. The next day, July 24, 1991, he attempted suicide. Thankfully, he was hospitalized before the rat poison killed him.

Terrence Luther Long was born in Columbia, South Carolina on July 21, 1959. After high school, he joined the military where he excelled at power weightlifting and football. In 1979, he attended Columbia Junior College to continue playing football. His talents were quickly recognized, and by 1980, he was playing on the line for West Carolina State. He continued weight training and was voted third strongest power lifter in the world. In 1983, he was considered the strongest college player in the United States. As a right guard, he was honored as a college All American. Terry was less than six feet tall and weighed 284 pounds.

Short the credits he needed for a degree in physical education, Long was chosen in the fourth round of the 1984 draft by the Pittsburgh Steelers as a right guard. He played eight consecutive seasons with the Steelers, some of those years alongside "Iron Mike" Webster.

In 1987, in a game against the Houston Oilers, Terry experienced a direct head-on hit. He was exhibiting classic signs of concussions and was admitted overnight to the hospital. Upon release, his play was restricted a week due to continuing confusion, light headedness, and difficulty concentrating. Although Terry confirmed to his wife that he had many "dings" to his head, he played through them.

In 1990, Long's SUV rolled over. When the police arrived they realized that he had lost consciousness. He, once again, experienced the classic symptoms of a severe concussion.

Although Long returned to play after his '91 steroid suspension, he tore a muscle in his right arm in his third game. He was not re-signed the following year.

After football, Terry endured surgeries on his knees, elbow, and shoulder. He knew the chronic pain associated with arthritis and the crippling effects of playing the offensive line. The other problems he suffered were subtle and known only to his wife and close friends. He became unreliable and impulsive. He started businesses on a whim without the review of a lawyer or any form of due diligence. He guaranteed business loans with his personal money. He was desperate but could not figure out what was going wrong. He felt everyone was out to get him and became agitated when he went out in public.

On March 29, 2005, Terrence Luther Long was indicted on federal charges of arson and bank fraud. Apparently, on the same day in 2003, that he filed Chapter 11 bankruptcy for Terry Long Enterprises, his chicken processing plant burned to ashes. The insurance settlement was $1.1 million.

Less than three months later, on June 7th, with his world in disarray, Terry Long drank anti-freeze and died. During the postmortem, Long was found to have Chronic Traumatic Encephalopathy. The result of the severe concussions he suffered while defending the Steelers's quarterback for eight years.

Bennet Omalu, MD, wrote in "Play Hard, Die Young":

"...analysis of Terry's brain confirmed the presence of gridiron dementia. There were large accumulations of abnormal proteins (tau protein) in tissues and cells throughout his brain. A significant number of his brain cells had died and disappeared...Regions of his brain responsible for mood, emotions, and executive functioning were all damaged by accumulated abnormal proteins"

Gridiron dementia or CTE is a result of brain trauma, and Long suffered two documented cases of severe concussions.

After retirement, Long professed that the National Football League had let him down. He had been a diligent player on the offensive line protecting the quarterback. He had destroyed his body for the Steelers. When Terry Long filed a worker's compensation claim with the NFLP layers Association for chronic pain and stiffness in his shoulders and knee joints, it was denied.

Suicide is dangerous if you fail, but Terry Long felt he had no choice.

A sure fire way to commit suicide is to place a gun to your head and pull the trigger. In the early morning hours of November 20, 2006, Andre Waters was pronounced dead in Tampa, Florida. He had owned a home in Hillsborough County, where he coached at the University of South Florida. He was a popular presence in a football crazed town. All football players were welcomed in Tampa, regardless of which team they represented.

Andre Waters was, in many ways, a hometown boy. He was born in 1962, in Belle Glade, more often than not referred to simply as south of "the lake" — meaning south of Lake Okeechobee. Belle Glade was a sleepy little town whose local restaurant was the gas station microwave and pre-packaged food. Andre's future would have been in the sugar cane industry, had he stayed. But he was determined to leave and find a way to provide for his mother and ten siblings. So Andre played high school football with a vengeance, determined to be noticed. His hard work was rewarded with a football scholarship to Cheney State University in Philadelphia. He became a member of the All-American Small College football team along with receiving his B.A. in business administration.

Due to his small size (5'11" and under 200 lbs.), Andre was overlooked in the 1984 draft. He signed, however, with the Philadelphia Eagles and after his first year, started at defensive back for eight years. He ended his National Football League career playing with the Cardinals in 1994 and '95.

To accommodate his small stature, Waters played hard. At one point he was nicknamed "Dirty Waters" for his low hits and aggressive play.

During the time he played football he suffered multiple concussions. More than once, his teammates had to direct him to the correct side of the field as he wandered toward the opposing team's bench. Not understanding the importance of symptoms such as headaches and blurred vision, Waters took a whiff of smelling salts and returned to the field to claim his position and job. His mother needed him. He'd bought her a house and provided for his brothers and sisters. He had to play.

When Andre left the NFL a cousin noticed his forgetfulness, confusion, and mood swings. Other relatives became concerned when Waters showed signs of severe depression. It's reported that at this time he attempted suicide with prescription medications and another attempt with carbon monoxide poisoning. His friends reported conversations with a paranoid Andre asking for help and wondering what was wrong.

But Andre couldn't break the cycle of physical pain due to the brutal blows his body took on the field, beginning in high school. He began relying on narcotics to dull the constant headaches and arthritic pain. His broken fingers and toes throbbed. Walking was excruciating.

He filed for disability under the NFL retirement plan, where his claim was denied. The National Football League used him, abused him, and threw him away. Understandably, he became very bitter.

Waters wanted to become an NFL coach but didn't have a mentor to smooth the way for him. He invested in a restaurant and pet grooming company as well as other ventures. Although he had a degree in business administration, he failed to research the investments, and he lost his money.

By 2006, along with his poor physical state and emotional instability, Waters was losing his cognitive abilities. He couldn't reason, and he couldn't figure out what was happening to him. He was no longer in control of his life. Sad and confused, Andre took to carrying his Bible with him. Then on November 20th, he was dead.

Dr. Omalu had this to say regarding the autopsy:

"brain sections revealed…abundant amounts of abnormal proteins that are typically found in the brains of eighty-plus-year old individuals who have a certain type of dementia, changes similar to those found in the brains of boxers who suffer from dementia pugilista or punch drunk syndrome."

At age forty-four, Andre Waters was returned to Belle Glade south of "the lake" for burial. He joined the growing ranks of those who lost their lives to gridiron dementia.

The articles following John Glenn Grimsley's death would have you believe he made a perfect transition to life after football. It was noted that he was in good health at age forty-five, and had a hunting and fishing expedition business.

He was happily married with two sons. His death on February 6, 2008, was an accident. He would never consider suicide. He was well-adjusted in retirement from the NFL

Grimsley was drafted in 1984 in the 6th round by the Houston Oilers. Out of the University of Kentucky, he proved to be a hard-hitting, hard-working lineman. His teammates and coaches were impressed with the effort he put into every hit. His play earned him a spot in the 1988 NFL Pro Bowl.

John was the epitome of the blue collar National Football League player. He did his job, he worked hard to condition his body, and he pursued ball carriers with vengeance. Then he quietly walked back to the huddle for his next assignment. He didn't brag or give flamboyant interviews. He was respectful and played the game without complaint or fanfare.

After seven seasons with the Oilers, Grimsley played with Dan Marino and the Dolphins for two years. After nine years of consecutive play, even John had no idea how many concussions he had suffered. He just continued doing his job.

On February 6, 2008, John cleaned his firearm for the last time. He died that morning of a gunshot wound. A post-mortem study of Grimsley's brain tissue showed damage consistent with chronic traumatic encephalopathy.

John Grimsley was not in good health, and he was not happy. He experienced the effects of gridiron trauma: depression, confusion, paranoid thoughts, and loss of control. He just wasn't going to admit it. He played tough and was uncomplaining on the football field, and that was the way he lived his life afterward.

Virginia, John's wife, had these words of advice, "The stigma needs to go away that you're a sissy if you come out of a game and don't go back in. A concussion is a big deal. It's not just a ding."

6

Yes, a Ding is Serious

When I was thirty-eight years old, I had a horseback riding accident. My horse was actually bucking with all four feet off the ground, and his back arched. My friends who witnessed this debacle said I fell about eight feet. My back hit first, and my head whip-lashed to the ground afterward. I was briefly unconscious. When I was roused, I saw these magnificent golden stars moving backward and forward on a deep navy blue background. I was entranced. However, nausea ensued, and the stars receded.

I took a few Tylenols and rested for awhile prone on a picnic table. After an hour, I drove my children and their friends ninety minutes back to Tampa. I rested for an hour and then realized I was in serious trouble. My left leg was completely numb, I couldn't stand without losing my balance, and I was vomiting from the pain. Most importantly, I realized I couldn't supervise four children. I called our team doctor.

The EMT's arrived. After a thorough examination at the hospital, I was told I had crushed lumbar discs four and five and was leaking spinal fluid. I had also snapped all of the transverse processes. My back looked on x-ray like a limp Christmas tree. I thought that was the worst of it. I was so wrong.

Many months later, it was discovered that I suffered a severe concussion in the fall. One doctor referred to it as a "brain shear." I had no balance. I couldn't shut my eyes, or I would fall over. To stay upright in the shower, I leaned against the cold tile walls. Interestingly, I was aphasic as well. When I tried to say "swimming pool," it came out as "water hole." Talk about frustrating! My friends would look at me in wonder as they watched their formerly erudite friend search for words.

One other subtle effect of the accident became obvious as I became more independent. Within three month after the shock of the accident subsided, I realized I had lost my ability to go back in time. In other words, if you asked me when I had my last dental appointment, I had no idea. It could have been a year or two days ago. This alarmed me. I realized for certain that I had cognitive damage when this symptom lasted over a year. Slowly, over a period of six months, the aphasia cleared, and I retrained my balance. However, over twenty-five years later, I still suffer brain damage from that concussion. It's as if you scrambled an egg but the shell remained intact. I didn't break my head, but I broke my brain.

To this day, I can't go back in time. I blew out the temporal part of my brain that processes past events. I live by way of hand-held time managers. I was the first of my friends to buy a Palm Pilot. Before that, I had calendars and appointment books. Yes, I have found ways to cope, but I know to avoid a second concussion...and my paycheck is not dependent on putting myself at risk for further concussions.

The Center for the Study of Traumatic Encephalopathy (CSTE) at Boston University School of Medicine defines CTE as "a progressive neurodegenerative disease caused by repetitive trauma to the brain...characterized by the build-up of a toxic protein called Tau on the form of neurofibrillary tangles (NFT's) and neuropil threads (NT's) throughout the brain. The abnormal protein initially impairs the normal functioning of the brain and eventually kills brain cells. Early on, CTE sufferers may display clinical symptoms such as memory impairment, emotional instability, erratic behavior, depression and problems with impulse control. However, CTE eventually progresses to full-blown dementia."

In his prepared remarks for the House Judiciary Committee concerning football-related head injuries, NFL Commissioner, Roger Goodell, wrote: "Recently, a number of media stories have been published about a condition known as CTE-chronic traumatic encephalopathy. As you may hear from other witnesses today, this condition has been seen in the brains of several former NFL players, in athletes in other sports, and even in an athlete who was only 18 years old. How susceptible athletes and others are to this condition and the precise causes and contributing factors, are issues for scientists and doctors to study and decide. It is fair to assume that head trauma MAY (my emphasis) play a role."

During his testimony, Linda Sanchez of California asked Goodell to read from the NFL handbook that football players are given:

Question: "If I have more than one concussion, am I at increased risk for another injury?"

Answer: "Current research with professional athletes has not shown that having more than one or two concussions leads to permanent problems if each injury is managed properly. It is important to understand that there is no magic number for how many how many concussions is too many."

It became apparent to those in the gallery that day and to the witnesses present that Roger Goodell was either poorly informed, had not read a paper in years, or he was deliberately obfuscating the truth. One began to wonder if he had read the NFL's own research. Which doctors had he been consulting who would mislead him in such a fashion?

On October 28, 2009, Dr. Eleanor Perfetto testified before the House Judiciary Committee chaired by the Honorable John Conyers. Her testimony held the room spellbound.

"My husband, Ralph Wentzel played as an offensive guard in the NFL for seven seasons. He retired in 1974 and became a high school-and college-level physical education teacher and football coach. In 1995 — over 20 years after his retirement from the NFL — my husband began having vague and disconnected symptoms: depression, general uneasiness and anxiety, always losing things like his wallet or checkbook. Today we recognize those symptoms as resulting from Chronic Traumatic Encephalopathy (CTE). In the following years, Ralph began to suffer obvious memory loss and confusion. In the fall of 1999, ten years ago, at the age of 56, Ralph was diagnosed with mild cognitive impairment, or MCI, a condition known to progress to Alzheimer's disease.

Ralph's condition did progress over the next ten years to full dementia related to CTE. I can't tell you on what day his condition flipped from MCI to dementia. However, in those 10 years, he lost his ability to work, drive a car, play golf, read the biographies he loved, cook gourmet meals, and enjoy a glass of wine. He can no longer dress, bathe, or feed himself. He lost his dry sense of humor. He lost his warm, quiet personality. He lost it all. Almost three years ago, I had to place my husband in an assisted living facility for dementia patients and he still resides there today. But frankly, my husband no longer has a life, certainly not one he'd want for himself."

"Repetitive trauma to the brain," what does that mean? That means that linemen going up against each other time and time again with an impact approaching fifteen hundred pounds and quarterbacks being thrown to the ground by men who then trample them.

Pro Football Hall of Fame quarterback Warren Moon says he had at least five concussions in his playing days. More specifically, his first concussion was at the age of eleven. Moon, now a spokesman for the Sports Concussion Institute, was quoted in *USA Today*, "There were a lot of other times of being dinged and seeing stars…and shaking it off. You never knew if you had a concussion or not because you did not allow yourself to stop."

In my own limited way, I understand not stopping. When I suffered a concussion, saw stars and was nauseated, no one ever told me these symptoms indicated brain injury. Cartoon characters saw stars every Saturday morning on television. They always got up and kept running. In *The Road Runner Show*, Wile E. Coyote fell off cliffs, saw stars, and kept up his pursuit.

I thought I was fairly well-informed—I'd worked in a medical school in child psychiatry, I read books and kept current on research. I certainly knew nothing about "seeing stars" as a dangerous signal.

I was so misinformed that following the Road Runner's example, I got back on the horse within minutes of my fall and rode another twenty minutes. I thought that was what I was supposed to do. "Get back on the horse." It never occurred to me to call 911 or stay off the horse. How could I be injured? I just pulled a muscle in my back and saw a few stars. I may have missed a few minutes of my life lying unconscious, but I didn't know it. Nothing ever happened to me. I was invincible; I was a cowgirl. I was the Road Runner.

We start telling our toddlers when they are learning to walk, "You're okay. Get back up. You can do this. Come to

Mommy." These children are trained early on to ignore pain and stay in pursuit of the goal. They get their initial praise from their parents. Later they'll get team congratulations and a bonus in their paychecks.

Although there is more publicity about concussions these days, there is little actual data as to how one identifies whether they have suffered one. Players such as Warren Moon refer to them as "dings." My car gets a "ding." But a dent is serious and I take it to a body shop. A player does not view a "ding" as serious. Blurred vision is a by-product of protecting your quarterback. One lineman I spoke with told me his teammates had to nudge him or guide him toward the man he was to block. My friend had his choice of ten men in his blurred vision field, but in reality, there was only one man he had to block.

Veteran player Troy Vincent had six documented concussions in the NFL but he guesses dozens more. He told *New York Times* reporter, Alan Schwarz, "Outside of me being knocked out, asleep, I went back in the game on all the other occasions. And 50 or 60 times, I'm in the huddle, I don't know where I'm at, don't know the call, and I've got a player holding me up. I'm not sure if athletes really know what a concussion is—get some smelling salts and get back in the game."

When you see one man lagging toward the huddle, he probably doesn't realize he is on a football field. "Hey, man, where am I?" isn't an uncommon question. These are not "dings." These are the after-shocks of brain trauma.

One of these concussions is bad. Two concussions equal more than one plus one in terms of brain damage. Three sends you into a different plane all together. The effects are cumulative. This is the repetitive head trauma that kills brain cells and leads to early onset of dementia. This is what caused the deaths of Terry Long, Mike Webster, Andre Waters, Tom McHale, Justin Grimsley and Justing Strzelczyk before they reached age fifty. Although Tom McHale never knowingly suffered a concussion, the 320 pound lineman suffered a conservative estimate of over twenty thousand hits to the head. His position and style of play on the line had the effect of a whiplash. As his hulking body slammed into the man in front of him, his head whipped forward, when he was stopped his head flipped backward. This had the effect of sending his brain crashing into his skull. Think shaken baby syndrome. Think Chronic Traumatic Encephalopathy.

Like Mike Webster, there are All-Pro players who are homeless. There are also many unknown players without a bed at night. We see them from afar, assuming they never worked, or are drug addicted, or crazy. We never assume a homeless man played in the National Football League.

Many contracts are built on incentives. The player reaches a certain goal and a bonus is paid. In order to receive that money, the player must stay in the game. If a quarterback needs to be sacked, one cannot do it sitting on the bench recovering from a headache. Additionally, a player does not want his back-up to have the opportunity to show the coaches he can play the position as well as the starter, if not better. Remember, there are very few guaranteed contracts in the NFL.

Players need their jobs. They are ill-prepared to begin a new career. It is incumbent upon them to keep their football job as long as possible. Therefore, even as one ages or plays with a broken body, to show weakness is to jeopardize your remaining career. A player cannot appear weak or vulnerable; the opposing team will take advantage of that fact and pummel the player out of the game. And...your teammates depend on you to fortify your position. The pervasive mentality is that you cannot let the team down.

However, the results of encouraging a player to return too soon may not have the desired results. As more researchers continued to study the cumulative negative effect of multiple concussions, we were given a living example by Pittsburgh Steelers quarterback Ben Roethlisberger. His latest concussion was his fourth documented concussion in five years of NFL play, including the one he sustained on his motorcycle. After a concussion on October 22, 2006, Roethlisberger returned to play the following week. In that game against Oakland, he threw four interceptions. The Raiders won the game.

Clearly, Roethlisberger was in no shape to return so early to play. It wasn't good for him or his team. But in 2006, this was standard operating procedure in the NFL. Concussions were not taken seriously. However, the effects of returning a player to the field before the concussion healed, didn't always work to the team's advantage. This was the culture at the time. Your teammates expected you to play, and your coaches expected you on the field on game day.

As if these factors aren't enough, players rarely have the cognitive abilities to know when to stop playing. Time and time again, players stay in the game too long. Their reflexes start to fail as they take more and more hits. These repetitive traumas to the brain make it impossible to assess ability or reasonableness for those players to remain in the National Football League. Oftentimes you will see a player taken out of the NFL by a father or a well-meaning relative. More often, a doctor will call a halt to a player's career.

Steve Young was arguably the Buccaneers' best quarterback. He certainly went on to prove that fact once he left our roster. For years I watched Steve get sacked or scramble for the sidelines. He was a committed player both on and off the field. Steve, a Mormon from Brigham Young

University, gave our team respect. He was well educated and soft-spoken and studied law in the off-season. And every time I watched him hit the ground, I winced.

Once, we almost lost Steve in a snow bank. We were in Green Bay, Wisconsin, in the winter. The Packers played us in the summer heat while we played them in the coldest part of the year. They had cleared the field of snow before the game. This created large snow banks on the sidelines. Unfortunately, it was still snowing, and Green Bay had chosen to wear dark green jerseys. The Buccaneers were, therefore, playing in white jerseys and white pants. Steve couldn't find a receiver, as they blended in with the falling snow. He took off running, ran out-of-bounds and dove into a snow bank. He didn't get up. He was stuck. Finally someone realized it and pulled Steve by the back of his jersey out of the snow. Our quarterback almost asphyxiated in front of a national audience.

Ray Perkins arrived, then Vinny Testaverde, and we reluctantly said good-bye to Steve Young. I followed his career and was pleased when he was elected to the Pro Football Hall of Fame. However, I was more proud of him for knowing when to leave the National Football League.

As Steve's career progressed, he suffered more head trauma. Standing in the pocket and being blind-sided time and again causes repetitive brain damage. Steve started to suffer more frequent documented concussions.

Meanwhile, Troy Aikman in Dallas was having the same problems. It was taking the Cowboys' quarterback longer for him to get up after being hit. His head was fuzzy and his thinking process was taking longer to re-orient. It was time.

Rarely will a player willingly exit the National Football League. Troy and Steve are wise men. Did they stay too long? Perhaps. Time will tell. Troy speaks openly of having migraine headaches now. Terry Bradshaw is another quarterback who left the game while his knees could still carry him. He recently came forward to discuss the residual symptoms of concussions that he is now experiencing. Meanwhile they set examples for other players to leave the game with dignity.

Within the past year, an eighteen year-old high school football player died. On autopsy his brain showed evidence or chronic traumatic encephalopathy. He is the youngest victim to date of this devastating condition. It was noted that he experienced multiple concussions in high school football.

Robert Stern, Ph.D., associate professor of Neurology and co-director of the Boston University School of Medicine Alzheimer's Disease Clinical and Research Program and co-director of the CSTE, stated, "CTE is the only fully preventable cause of dementia...meaningful guidelines (need) to be implemented at all levels of athletic participation, from youth to college to pro. In the meantime, however, we already know that return to play too soon after a concussion can have devastating results."

But for younger players, whether high school or college, they follow in the footsteps of their heroes. Super Bowl February, 2009, Steelers' quarterback Ben Roethlisberger played after suffering a spinal cord concussion on December 28, 2008. Lying motionless on the turf at Heinz Stadium, Roethlisberger admitted to reporter Gerry Dulac that it was scary when "that special look passed between the team doctor and the trainer." After fifteen long minutes, during which Roethlisberger could not feel pins being inserted into his arms, he was transferred on a special spinal board to a hospital noted for its brain institute. Although he was released within twenty-four hours, Roethlisberger's headaches did not clear for several days.

Unfortunately, this incident marked the third time Roethlisberger experienced a severe concussion. Just before pre-season in 2006, he was in a motorcycle accident. Riding without a helmet, Ben suffered a concussion and additionally had to have his appendix removed. Later that season, in a game against the Atlanta Falcons, he had his second concussion.

According to Judy Batista of the *New York Times*, Ben is known as a player who "plays through injuries" whether concussions or shoulder problems. As Roethlisberger said about his third documented concussion, "We are putting all that in the past and moving on." Interestingly, Ben didn't seem to learn anything from last season. He began the 2009 season suffering further concussions. The man never wanted to take a break. In week eleven he suffered a concussion. However, he continued to practice with the team the entire week. On Thursday he boasted that he had a better baseline (cognitive functioning) score than prior to the beginning of the season. In his estimation, he was in perfect form to play three days hence, so he continued to practice.

However, that week the NFL decided to come down strongly on concussed players being allowed to take the field too early, and Ben was benched. Teammate Hines Ward was vocal in the news outlets and stated that he couldn't understand allowing Roethlisberger to practice all week long only to pull him off the field the day before the game. Ward thought Ben should force the issue. He noted that he oftentimes got around the rules by lying to his coaches or team doctors. Ward believed the team was more important than individual players.

For the millions of youth players, what message does this Super Bowl winning quarterback send? In 2007, Alan Schwarz, *New York Times* reporter interviewed Matt Lohr, a high school quarterback in western Pennsylvania, this question.

"(Lohr) played through a concussion last year and experienced months of memory and cognitive problems that affected his homework. Lohr played

in a green no. 4 jersey—the same as his hero, the
Packers' Favre—and later admitted that doing as
Mr. Favre did was his mantra: 'Sure,' Lohr said, 'His
whole thing was playing through pain.'"

Schwarz further writes:

> "Experts say the most frustrating aspect of
> concussions in football is the silence surrounding
> them. Football's play-with-pain mentality discourages
> players from high school to the pros from revealing
> this virtually imperceptible injury to coaches or
> trainers, often causing more serious harm."

Kelly Jasmon, a high school senior with three documented
concussions also spoke with Alan Schwarz in his September 15,
2007, *New York Times* article, "Silence on Concussions Raises
Risks of Injuries." When asked if he sustained another
concussion this season would he tell a coach or trainer, Kelly
responded, "No chance. It's not dangerous to play with a
concussion. You've got to sacrifice for the sake of the team. The
only way to come out is on a stretcher."

What seventeen or eighteen year old has the medical
expertise to make these decisions? Most professional players
cannot accurately describe a concussion. High school coaches are
not trained sufficiently to understand the harm generated on
immature brains. Trainers are a rarity on the sidelines of high
school games. Certified. trainers do not factor into most
educational budgets. The idea of a high school team physician or
neurologist is a laughing matter. So where the risk of trauma is
the greatest, the medical resources are basically non-existent.

On the Buccaneers' sideline, our team physician was a
general surgeon. We had an orthopedist on the sideline as

well. Where was a neurologist? He was in the stands with a pager on his belt. Since the most severe injuries usually involve the brain, wouldn't it make sense to require a neurologist on the sideline alongside the team physician?

However, with the swelling sizes of college players and crushing blows in high school games, neurologists should be required on the sidelines of these games as well. At this point, physicians and certified trainers are no-shows at high school and Pop Warner games. It is well understood that brains continue to mature as the child grows physically.

A teenage brain is not fully mature. Therefore, it is susceptible to trauma at a higher rate than that of a college player whose brain resembles that of a pro-player. Just as a severe injury to a seventeen year-old's knee can sideline his career, a hit that crashes his brain against his skull can end his career and leave him with poor cognitive processing including depression, memory loss, and fuzzy thinking. This combined with severe headaches makes concussions worth taking seriously. As Robert Sallis, president of the American College of Sports Medicine told *New York Times'* Alan Schwarz, "Poor management of high school players' concussions isn't just a football issue. It's a matter of public health."

It is a medical fact that the skulls of females close and solidify at age eighteen, which is two years after males. This puts girls' brains at significant risk for concussions.

Since girls are rarely found on the football field, their injuries primarily occur on the soccer field. Girls' soccer has exploded in popularity since the early 70s when Title IX was passed. This legislation mandated equality and equal opportunity for girls' sports within the federally funded education system. While football was king, using the majority of school funds to support scholarships and playing costs, schools and universities now had to provide comparable services for girls' teams.

Girls' soccer, baseball, basketball, volleyball, and softball blossomed in high school and college campuses. With the Olympic wins by women's teams representing the United States, interest in women's sports soared. Mia Hamm became an idol to teenage girls and put girls' soccer on the map.

Swept up in this tide of enthusiasm was a young girl from a small town in Massachusetts. Kate started playing soccer in middle school. She was a standout player. Lithe and quick, her feet moved like a dancer's. She was everywhere and fearless in her efforts to reach the ball. Kate headed the ball with abandon. There was little to hold back in her enthusiastic play – certainly no protective gear.

The first concussion she suffered occurred when she and an opponent tried to head the ball simultaneously. Both fell to the ground. Kate was unconscious. For several minutes the stadium was soundless. Kate roused with the help of her high school coach and was led to the bench. In the early years of this century, no one thought about being headed by an opponent. This was part of the game. Kate reported headaches and dizziness to her parents that continued for several days. Her parents thought that these symptoms would resolve shortly. They did not pick up on the warning signs of a concussion.

Kate returned to school and soccer practice the following day. She was on the Dean's List and didn't want to jeopardize her academic future of going to college to become a nurse. Kate's teachers encouraged her. The fact that she was a star on the soccer team would be a plus on her college application.

During her senior year, Kate put pressure on herself to achieve perfect grades. Along with this goal, she was determined to have her team reach the championship game.

Unfortunately, in striving to be the best, Kate suffered another on-field concussion. This too, was the result of her aggressive play. She and her opponent headed each other instead of the ball, frontal lobe to frontal lobe without the benefit of a helmet. Kate was out and on the ground, unresponsive to those surrounding her.

Not knowing the devastating effects of a second concussion, Kate was seated on the bench when she became conscious. The next day she was at school sporting a knot on her forehead and a blazing headache. Neither her coach nor her parents were aware of the seriousness of what was occurring inside Kate's brain.

Five years later, Kate's parents contacted me. Kate was twenty-three years old and failing out of her nursing program. During this time, I was working pro bono as a parent/student advocate. Having a doctorate in special education, I am well-versed in the federal guidelines for ancillary services for students with special needs.

Having been friends with Kate's family for many years, I suggested a third party psychologist evaluate Kate's intelligence and achievement potential on a battery of tests.

When I received the report, I was devastated. I called the psychologist and asked if Kate had mentioned anything about being hit on the head or suffering concussions. She confirmed with me that Kate had, by her admission, suffered at least two concussions. I called the parents for confirmation. Yes, she had been knocked unconscious twice while playing soccer in high school.

The test results showed scores in the genius range, Kate's former functioning in school. The scores also showed severe short term memory loss, Kate's present level of functioning. Her below-normal scores outnumbered her above-normal results.

I met with her parents and explained what I thought had happened. I described the effects of the toxin Tau which was probably released into her brain on the second impact/concussion. I explained that Kate would in the future, if not now, suffer depression that could not be treated by psychotropic drugs or talk therapy.

I described the chaos that goes on in an emergency room, where memory is all a nurse has time for in treating a number of patients simultaneously. I walked them through their last doctor's visit where they were one of five patients in cubicles, how the nurse was in charge of keeping straight - who had what problem. Every scenario required the nurse to use her short term memory.

Kate had no short term memory. How was she going to keep the diagnoses and the patients' treatments plans in her head? She had no time to dictate or write herself notes. Being a nurse is memory dependent. These cognitive deficits were causing her to flunk out of nursing school.

Even if I could find ancillary services to aid Kate in completing the nursing program, I could not recommend that she become a nurse.

I explained the legal complications to her parents. Knowing Kate had these intellectual losses, who would knowingly place her in the position of possibly harming patients in her care? I asked them the ultimate question, "Would you want Kate to be *your* nurse?"

I described Kate's future. Besides depression, she would most likely experience early onset dementia; her personality might morph into someone they no longer knew. She might resort to heavy use of pain medication to quiet the severe headaches she will suffer. Ultimately she will most likely require an assisted living facility.

When looking at the psychologist's test results, I knew in an instant Kate was suffering the effects of concussion damage. Tau had been released into her brain. At twenty-three years of age, Kate's future was pre-determined. The symptoms of a deteriorating brain were only going to increase. Her parents are shocked. How could soccer have such a life altering effects? It's only a game: a game for girls. Football is dangerous; violence is the premise of that game.

It is clear parents and coaches need to take soccer seriously. These injuries have lasting, devastating effects. Kate is not the only young woman to experience the catastrophic results of concussions on the field.

I believe it is time to prohibit heading the ball in all games below the college level. Let's give our girls a chance to live their professional dreams as women without intellectual deficits.

In an interview on CNN January 31, 2009, Sanjay Gupta, M.D., was revisiting the issue of concussions and football with Dr, Ann McKee, co-director of the Center for the Study of Traumatic Encephalopathy and an associate professor of neurology and pathology at the Boston University School of Medicine. The Super Bowl was less than a week away and all eyes were on Ben Roethlisberger and Kurt Warner. Their histories of concussions were making bookies nervous. But more to the point, concussions were finally getting the notice they deserved. Concussions are dangerous, more dangerous than a broken throwing arm or dislocated shoulder. The following is an excerpt of Gupta's on air discussion with McKee.

January 28, 2009
CNN News Transcript: January 29, 2009

Announcer: All concussions have one thing in common: they temporarily interfere with how your brain works. Any bump to the head can cause a concussion. But some people are at higher risk than others, for example athletes who participate in contact sports. And once you've had a concussion, doctors say you're more likely to have others. Dr. Sanjay Gupta explores the possible consequences.

GUPTA: A new study confirms what some scientists have long suspected: concussions start an injury cascade......

MCKEE: I think what's been surprising is that it's so extensive. It's throughout the brain, not just on the superficial aspects of the brain, but it's also deep inside.

GUPTA: This is a healthy brain, and this is the brain of a former NFL player in his 40s. Those brown tangles, those indicate brain damage that can eventually kill cells. The trauma in this NFL player's brain looks a lot like damage in this brain, a 70 year old who suffered from dementia.
(See Fig. 1)

GUPTA: Did it surprise you to see some of these things?

MCKEE: Oh, absolutely, absolutely. To see the kind of changes we're seeing in forty-five year olds is basically unheard of.

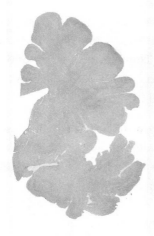 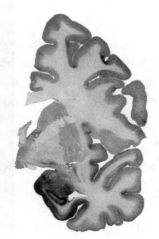

HEALTHY BRAIN   **FORMER NFL PLAYER**

MCKEE: I think the message is that we need to identify what constitutes a significant head injury and we need to treat it sufficiently, and I think that probably means resting an injury a lot more than we rest it.

GUPTA: You're a neurologist.

MCKEE: Right.

GUPTA: I'm a neurosurgeon. I think it'd be fair to say that concussions are still a somewhat vaguely diagnosed thing, right?

MCKEE: Absolutely.

GUPTA: What is a concussion?

MCKEE: It could be a sense of fogginess or being dazed or seeing stars or it can be a loss of consciousness. A concussion was defined as "the absence of physical damage to the brain." There's no bruising of the brain. There's no hemorrhage into the brain. You do a CT Scan, you don't see anything, was there a concussion, there's no skull fracture.

But I think what we're discovering now is that concussion is a microscopic injury. And it's a metabolic injury. And it's -- we see changes in axons and changes to the nerve cells that are occurring at a much more microscopic level.

GUPTA: What is the message of the research then?

MCKEE: Well, I think, you know, if we can just draw attention to the fact that multiple traumas, concussive, probably sub-concussive injuries sustained over an individual's lifetime, but probably, more importantly, sustained in early adulthood, can lead to a progressive neurologic deterioration that appears to show up in their midlife.

We think it starts at a time that they have these repeated traumas and it sort of starts to trigger a cycle that sort of go -- progresses but is undetected until 10, even 20 years later when they come down with some behavioral changes, memory loss, depression, and actually the beginnings of this chronic neurodegenerative change -- the beginnings (ph).

GUPTA: College athlete right now...

MCKEE: Right.

GUPTA: ...or high school athlete even, if they're watching this or their parents are watching it and they may have had a concussion. What would you -- what would you tell them?

MCKEE: I would tell them to take it very seriously. I would tell you, not only to take it very seriously but make sure it gets a lot of rest. And I think, personally, they all need at least a month of rest after a concussion.

The experts have spoken. Will we follow their advice? Let's hope so for our children and our grandchildren.

When I try to search for a safe sport it is like an oxymoron. Are there any safe sports? My father played golf. He was hit twice with an errant ball. The first one hit him in the head, which required stitches and could have caused a concussion. The second time hit him squarely in the chest, over his heart. We were lucky he had a strong heart. The hospital personnel were only too happy to regale my father with stories of crazy golf balls zooming in irregular paths to hit an unsuspecting player. So much for safe.

So how about swimming? Seems safe enough. However, Roger Goodell's brother (yes, the commissioner of the National Football League) received a concussion while swimming. Apparently he hit the end of the pool with his head probably during a flip-turn gone awry. A freak accident, to be sure. But they do happen.

In January of 2011, American Olympian skier Lindsay Vonn crashed during a practice run. She suffered a concussion and was unable to compete for several weeks. She was quoted as saying that she could ski through pain but she couldn't ski with the after effects of a concussion.

I have collided with my opponent on the racquetball court where we have both gone out for the count. Fortunately neither of us could remember who caused what, as the game is so fast. I think the same could be said for handball. Crashing into walls and floors often leads one's head to be hit in the process: concussion time.

Basketball doesn't get a free pass, either. Along with soccer, basketball is a leading cause of concussions. Skulls are not fully formed until age eighteen, so there is plenty room for danger. It's a game of speed and sudden stops. It seems innocent enough until you consider how quickly their brain hit the front of the skull and ricochets off the back of the skull. Running down the court at full speed, momentum builds for a dangerous impact when the forward movement stops suddenly. It does not matter whether you are wearing Becky Harmon's jersey, Maya Moore's or another favorite player's, the magical power of your star's jersey will not save your brain.

At this stage of my life, it's difficult to get excited about any sport because I know the dangers and the backstory all too well. And it's not just with the game itself, but the equipment.

The selling of sports merchandise is often dependent upon the fact that a talented athlete wears a certain brand. The idea is that if you or your child wears that brand, you, too, will have the prowess of that player. As adults, we realize that it takes many years of hard work and practice to reach even half the ability most athletes' posses. But our kids don't believe that for a minute. Instead, our kids are bombarded with ads for shoes, tee shirts, and sports equipment. They want what their favorite athlete's shoes, bat, ball, racket, or helmet because they are convinced they will play just as well as their favorite athlete.

Helmets have no special powers. Unfortunately when a player straps on a helmet, he thinks his head is invincible. His parents don't realize there are differences among helmets. I have watched parents outfit their son for the upcoming football season by walking into local sports stores and choosing the cheapest helmet. Other common mistakes parents make are when they pass down a big brother's helmet or intentionally buy a larger size to last a few seasons by stuffing socks in the helmet to make it fit more snuggly.

Pop Warner Football and other community leagues have a fairly unscientific way of distributing their equipment. The helmets are placed in a pile, and the kids pick out the coolest helmet, the one with a visor or a special stripe or face guard. It has nothing to do with the fit. Unfortunately the coaches and parents don't appreciate or understand the need for a proper fit. If there's a helmet on a child's head, he must be imbued with powers to keep him safe.

The reason for this attitude is that parents and coaches assume that safety standards are maintained when manufacturing helmets. The regulatory agency: the National Operating Committee on Standards for Athletic Equipment (Nocsae) uses the same guidelines for professional and children's helmets and has not changed their requirements in decades. As recent research has proven that concussions are occurring at an alarming rate, the committee has been slow to act in enforcing tougher guidelines. Funded by the sporting goods industry, Nocsae has an inherent conflict of interest. New Mexico Senator, Tom Udall, has requested that the Consumer Products Safety Commission involve itself in the creation of newer standards. Clearly regulation by the industry itself is not lessening concussions and improving safety.

What parent thinks of this when her son takes the field? If a helmet is sold as head protection, they assume it will insure the brain against injury. Likewise, bike helmets, horseback riding helmets, skateboarding helmets, ski helmets, etc. Do they offer the false sense of security from harm?

Interestingly, a colleague of mine asked a local community football league of they'd like our organization to address their parents on safety issues of football. The administrator of the league declined, saying they had had a doctor address the group several years ago, and he had scared the parents. So, no, he did not want us to interfere with his parents because he feared losing players. Parents can't make informed choices for their children if the league won't allow the information to be distributed. Their goal is to keep the parents in the dark as to the dangers of the game.

7
Richard Wood:
The Fan's Favorite Blue Collar Worker

"Come on, Richie, you gotta play with us. Get your brother to take you to register," his friends said repeatedly. Bowing to peer pressure, nine-year-old Richard Wood, the youngest of nine children, asked his brother, Walter, to take him to sign up for little league baseball. "That was my first escapade into sports," he recalls.

Everybody played sports back then—no matter their background, neighborhood, ethnicity, or race. It was what children did in the late 1950s and early 1960s in the Northeast. And it was no different in Elizabeth, New Jersey, where the little boy with five sisters and three brothers grew up under the watchful eyes of his large family and his mother's ten siblings, almost all who lived nearby.

Children were sent outdoors to play when they weren't in school, doing homework, or chores. It was there in the sunshine that they learned to play sports on their own—in the streets, on the playgrounds, and at the schoolyards, wherever they could find the space for makeshift bases or, in the case of football, improvised goal posts. They could play just as long as they liked, but they had better be home before dark.

After school one day, while Rich, then ten, sat on the floor watching TV, his brother-in-law, Arnie Highsmith, a policeman who was active with the Police Athletic League (PAL), walked into the living room. "Richie, you're going to play football this year."

"I don't want to play any football," Rich responded.

"Yes, you are," his brother-in-law told him.

"So, the next thing I know," Rich said when recalling the story to me, "I'm doing side hops and push-ups because my brother-in-law wanted me to." It is this man who Richard attributes his lifelong involvement in football and his love of the game.

But it wasn't without challenge from the get-go. Police Lieutenant White, the PAL coach for Rich's team and his best friend's older brother, called him aside after his first training season. "You know, Richie," he said, sadly, "you're not going to make it this year."

Rich was so disappointed that he didn't try out for football the next year. The year after, when he was twelve, he made a second attempt at the PAL football team. But Rich's mother told him to take his uniform back. "She didn't want me to play football." So, obediently, he returned the uniform and quit the team before getting a chance to wear it.

It was when he was in the seventh grade that she finally acquiesced, and Richard Wood officially began playing organized football. He played in junior high and throughout his years at Thomas Jefferson High School, where he was no ordinary guard.

In his senior year, he was named All County as an offensive lineman for leading his team to two State titles. "I was being recognized as a good football player," he said, modestly.

Growing up during the Vietnam War and Civil Rights era and having two brothers who were twenty-year Air Force veterans, Rich thought about joining the military. "But, my family just encouraged me to do the things I wanted to do and to get a good job." Going to college or playing professional football never crossed his mind. However, his teammates and high school coaches encouraged him to continue academically.

"It was my best friend, who went on to play for the University of Michigan, who really persuaded me to pursue going to college on a football scholarship," Richard said. And, so it happened.

Colleges and universities in Michigan, Nebraska, Pennsylvania, and West Virginia beckoned. So did others including Rutgers, Montclair State, Maryland, and Ohio State — schools closer to home. Rich chose the University of Southern California (USC) which seemed a million miles away to many of his friends. They told him that he wouldn't make it that far from home.

"But I didn't have any detractors in my family," Richard said. He remembers his father, who worked at a General Motors plant in New Jersey for thirty years, telling him as he was about to leave home for California, "Just work hard, son. Do the best you can do, and that's all they can ask of you."

His family had a great deal of confidence in him. So in 1971, at age seventeen, the little boy who had not wanted to play *any* football when he was ten, went off to Los Angeles on a football scholarship. He was by then a strapping 6' 2" tall and 215 pounds. Bearded, he looked much older than his teammates.

His first night at USC, the freshmen team got together at Julie's, a famous restaurant then located across the street from the university, for an informal get-together. He had never met any of these young men before. "Our coach had us introduce ourselves," Rich said, "asking us to give our names, positions, and any honors received. But, before they did that, the coach asked that each of them share a joke to break the ice."

When it was his turn, Richard said, "I am Batman from Gotham City," a reference to the comic strip super-hero character who fiercely defended his city against crime. "They called me Batman from that night on," Rich said, because he was a violent fellow, and Batman was associated with crime fighting and violence. "When I play football, I'm a different person," he explained. "But I'm a nice person when I'm not."

He attributes his game demeanor in part to the great football movies he saw growing up, Knute Rockne and Jim Thorpe—*All American*, and others—and to all those black and white World War II movies, to the Vietnam War news stories, and to all that "you-gotta-be-strong, you-gotta-be-macho" mentality prevalent during the time. "You know," he said, "you can't cry. You have to accept pain. That was our direction."

Although it was difficult to be so far away from home and family, Richard enjoyed his USC experience. As a spectator at his first Trojans game, he met Karen, who would one day become his wife and the mother of his two children. "We played Alabama that day," he recalls, associating their meeting with the competition on the field. "I'll never forget it," he said.

Rich led the Trojans in tackles his sophomore and junior years. As a sophomore in 1972, he made five interceptions and one hundred twenty-nine tackles, winning USC's Player of the Game Award in a game against UCLA. He was chosen 1973 Playboy Pre-Season All-American, played in the 1973, 1974, and 1975 Rose Bowls, and in the 1975 Hula Bowl, Senior Bowl, and College All-Star Game. He served as USC squad captain in 1974.

Most notably, Richard Wood was selected All-American Linebacker in 1972, 1973, and 1974, becoming USC's first— and only—three-time All-American Linebacker in the school's long football history.

What he was most proud of, however, was being a member of the first freshmen class to go undefeated at home all four years. The Trojans won National Championships in

1972 and 1974. Both he and the team were named All Conference in 1972, 1973, and 1974. During his football career at USC, the Trojans won thirty-one games, tied two, and lost only two. His coach, John McKay, became one of Richard's role models.

It was confusing—and a personal let-down—that Rich was selected in the third round of the 1975 NFL draft by the New York Jets. He'd expected to be picked up in the first round. "It was disrespectful," he said, "because I had been on a team that won two national championships, was never injured, and played every game from high school through college. I knew I should have gotten higher up in the draft." But Richard was told that at 230 pounds, he was considered small for a linebacker.

That said, he was still considered among the top one hundred players in the country. "There are some ten million students playing football and only 1,600 of them get into the NFL. And I was one of them. I was walking on Cloud Nine, getting a chance to play at home and with Joe Namath."

As devoted as he was to the Jets and to helping the team win, Batman was traded after his first season. "The rumor was that they felt I was injury-prone, but I'd never been injured to where I couldn't play in a game."

During his second year in training camp, however, Richard was hit from behind. A 270-pound player rolled up on the back of his leg and he fell backwards, badly twisting and spraining his ankle and causing him to miss a couple of pre-season games.

At that time, there were six pre-season games, not four, as is the case now. But he felt he had enough time to heal before the season officially began. The Jets disagreed. Richard Wood was traded for a seventh round pick to the Tampa Bay Buccaneers.

Once again, he dismissed the disappointment of his NFL draft status. "That was just an ego thing," he said.

Richard joined the Buccaneers in 1976, the first year of play as an NFL expansion team. Heartened to again be playing for John McKay, his USC coach, Richard "Batman" Wood looked at his new assignment as a blessing. "Well, okay, I have an opportunity with a brand new team in the league to show how good I am and what they will miss in New York."

Although the team's first two seasons were horrible by anyone's standards, Rich did what his father told him to do when he went off to USC — do the very best that he could. Batman did just that and played with his heart, soul, and body.

He served as team captain in 1979, the year he made a career high one hundred fifty-eight tackles, including eighteen tackles in a National Football Conference Championship game against the Rams. The Bucs then had the league's top-rated defense, and a local paper named Rich the "Most Overlooked and Under-Rated Buc." The title fit.

In 1979, 1981 and 1982, the Bucs won its division and made the playoffs. Rich was an integral part of its celebrated defense. Considered one of the greatest linebackers in the team's history, Richard had five seasons with more than one hundred tackles and led the club in stops during four of them. He intercepted nine passes, caused twelve fumbles and scored three defensive touchdowns – ranking him as a fifth-place tie in club history. Batman Wood was the team's all-time leading tackler through the late 1990's with eight hundred fifty-five stops.

A fierce but popular player during his nine seasons with the Bucs, Rich played a key role in the club's turnaround during the late 70s and early 80s, when, much to the chagrin of the NFL, he was also well known for drawing or pasting bat insignias on his uniform hip, elbow and hand pads, on his socks and shoes, on the back of his helmet, and on the hand towel that hung from his belt.

When he left the Bucs in 1984, Rich had played in one hundred thirty-two games, a team record. He had started in eighty-nine, with eighty-eight of them consecutive games. Although he had recorded one hundred forty tackles in 1981, he was demoted to reserve status the following season, quite possibly because of a contract dispute. He had only one start in the next forty-one games and was released in 1984, even though according to him, he had never once — not one time — missed a game because of injury.

Rich wished they had traded him instead of keeping him on as an insurance policy, as a backup player. It was that coaching decision that likely fed the rumors that Rich may have been too injured to play. He thought the opposite.

In 1985, Richard "Batman" Wood ended his professional football career after playing one season with the Jacksonville Bulls of the United States Football League.

At thirty-three years old, after playing football for two-thirds of his life, he needed to make a transition away from the sport he loved. "We were taught how to prepare for football," he said. "Nobody ever taught us how to prepare for life *after* football."

8

How the Game Should Be Played

For the first time in his life, Richard floundered. During the next few years, he served as a part-time high school coach, gas station owner/operator, brewery worker, car salesman, and substitute teacher. On the side, Rich, a third-degree black belt in Tae Kwon Do, continued to practice his martial arts, as he had done each day throughout his football career.

It was Tae Kwon Do that gave him the focus, mental, and physical strength needed to make him an outstanding player. Now that his playing days were over, he thought about opening a Tae Kwon Do school and competing in the Olympics, but found neither idea ultimately viable.

He drove his beloved drag racing car, naming his personal Batmobile the Gotham City Special. But knew that was not where his future lay.

Richard missed football. And the fans missed him back. In a 1988 poll conducted by the St. Petersburg Times, Batman was voted among the top ten Bucs players of all time—and he hadn't played for the club in four years.

His patience paid off. In early 1991, at age thirty-seven and while recuperating from Achilles' tendon surgery, he received a welcome phone call. Bucs coach Richard Williamson had added Richard to his coaching staff as a defensive assistant and strength and conditioning coach. He was retained by Sam Wyche when Wyche took over from Williamson in 1992. However, two years later, Wyche let him go.

It made little sense. One popular sports columnist had, not long before, described Richard as a remarkable and durable athlete, a man who always talked of doing his best for the team and the fans, not for himself. Tom McEwen wrote that "quickness, football smarts, conditioning and want-to were his strengths." The writer also pointed out that Rich had never been involved in any mischief and was a model team player.

Sentiment was that he ought to have been better rewarded instead of being thrown away.

Richard was unlike players who got into drugs, caused trouble, or were arrested for violence or other crimes. "I was happy to have my family, my car, my martial arts — all the outlets I needed." He maintained that most other players didn't have all of that, and it caused them problems. "That's why I always admired Lee Roy Selmon, Rickie Bell, Derrick Brooks, and other guys who had other things going on besides football."

"Me, I'm a dinosaur." Richard just wanted to coach and teach.

Disappointed but resolute, Richard looked for other coaching opportunities. In 1994, he became head coach with the semi-pro Amsterdam Crusaders of the American Football Federation-Netherlands, taking the team to the playoffs. In 1995, he served as defensive assistant in the first Black College All Star Game. In 1996, he was honored at the Hula Bowl of Fame. And, in 1997, he coached the pro football Munich Cowboys of the German Football League.

He returned to Tampa from Europe in late 1997 and worked as a security resource officer for the local school district, assigned mostly to programs targeting dropout prevention. In 1998, he signed on as a defensive coordinator for a relatively new high school football team, the Wharton Wildcats. Shortly after, he was asked to take over as interim head coach.

Rich accepted even though he'd been offered coaching contracts with the German Amateur League and the European Federation Cup. A family man of the first order, Richard wanted to be closer to home, to his wife and his then-teenaged children. Besides, he saw the challenge in developing a high school team from almost scratch, with no area feeder school, a zero win record, and an enormous problem recruiting players.

The man who had placed number nine in a 1998 Buccaneer Magazine survey of the fifty greatest Bucs players of all times, wanted these young players to know what winning and what life was all about.

So slowly but surely, Rich began turning things around for the Wildcats. In 1999, the school conducted a search for a permanent coach. In competition with a field of widely-known former players and coaches, Rich was the one selected.

It was a decision backed by his players and their parents. It paid off as he led the team to an eventual 9-1 record and a shot at the state championship in 2002, the year that he was also named the Buccaneers "Coach of the Year," an award reserved for coaches who transformed their charges into high-potential football players and who made an impact on their team, school, and community.

That same year, he was voted — by coaches from around the state — as the Florida Dairy Farmers Coach of the Year. He was also named All-Suncoast Coach of the Year by The St. Petersburg Times.

In the fall of 2002, Rich was elected into the prestigious USC Hall of Fame at a ceremony at the Los Angeles Coliseum. Considered a star player in college, he had logged eleven years without missing a game as a sure-tackling linebacker.

In 2003, he coached the defensive line for NFL Europe's Frankfurt Galaxy and won his first championship ring when his team prevailed in the World Bowl XI. Frankfurt then led the league in rushing defense and was second in sacks.

Richard Wood was inducted into the 2007 National Football Foundation & College Hall of Fame. Described as "a fierce tackler and team leader," he then joined twenty-six other former Trojans who had made it into the College Football Hall of Fame.

Receiving these many honors and coaching a high school team to a state championship pleased him, but Richard was most proud that, in his five years as their coach, not one of his Wildcats had been seriously injured.

That was certainly not the case for so many other players.

As a player and a coach, Richard had seen a great many injuries. One of the worst happened when he played high school football. Rich was running a play back on the kick-off team and blocked an opposing player by hitting him high. He didn't see that one his teammates had also hit the same player low. "I just blocked him and then turned around and saw him on the ground. My teammate was screaming with excitement, 'I got him. I got him.' He was making a big deal out of it and laughing about it."

Later in the locker room, Coach VonBischoffhausen told Rich, who was then a team captain, to go see the boy he had blocked. "They're taking him to the hospital, and you should talk to him."

It turned out that the player who had hit him low had hit him in his leg and his bone was coming out of the side of his leg at a 90-degree angle. "It was a compound fracture. I felt so bad. I told him how sorry I was, that I was sure he'd be okay. And, I told my teammate that it wasn't right to cheer about it."

From that point on, Richard never made a big deal out of a hit and never celebrated a block during which someone had been injured. And he never thought much of the "kill, kill, kill" mentality coming from the stands.

He saw the same type of injury years later in a Bucs' game when defensive lineman Randy Crowder was simultaneously hit high and low. "His leg went sideways and he was just screaming. He couldn't move. He was like a turtle that had been turned upside down."

He explains that injury and pain are two different things in football. "Injury, like a broken leg sticking out at a 90-degree angle, may prevent you from playing. Pain, on the other hand is something you will have — and still play."

This is the nature of the game.

"Yes, in a way," he said. "It was my job to try my best to separate the opposing team from the ball. Yes, I am going to hit someone, but I'm going to hit him legally. I'm going to let them know that they're in a physical football game because I'm a physical football player, a violent linebacker. I wanted to be like Dick Butkus, Willie Lanier, and Ray Nitschke. I wanted to be one of the best that ever played this doggone game. But I would never gloat."

Others did, which bothered Rich a great deal. "They gloated big time. It's a man thing, a macho thing. You have to remember that when I was growing up, coaching was different than it is today. You can't walk up to kid in a football practice now and grab him by his helmet and slap him upside his head and say, 'What are you crying for?' You can't kick him or grab him by his face mask."

As Rich explains it, these were training methods used to make players tougher, just like the military did. Many coaches were former military or police, and they used some of that training when they coached football. "If you read stories about Bear Bryant and Texas A&M, you'll understand how they made you tough. How they made you forget the pain you had to go through. The sweat. The bleeding. The coaches would say, 'What are you worrying about that cut for? Put a band-aid on it and get back out there. What are you crying for?'"

But, it's different today. "You had better not do that to a young child – an eight, nine, or ten-year-old today. You can't grab a young boy and kick him. You can't grab his helmet. You can't slap him upside the head."

You can, however, better condition them so that they won't get hurt as much.

"When I was young," he said, "you weren't as conditioned. In college, we had only twenty days of spring training. We didn't have weight-lifting, running, and off-season conditioning programs like many schools now have." Better conditioning, Richard believes, translates into less injury.

Not to mention better coaching. "Youth coaches should have to get certified. They ought to be taught better ways to teach the game to the players. Make it more about technique than brute force."

Richard made sure that he coached differently than he had been coached.

"I think I was more of a teacher and organizer. More compassionate to the players because I knew what it was like to play, to practice every day, and have constantly on your mind how you would play during the next game. I had experienced it and knew what the players were going through. I knew about their personal lives and their families, too."

Richard made a committed effort to know his players because he felt that a personal touch was missing in his USC experience. "I never wanted them to feel like they were being thrown away when they were no longer able to play."

He made certain, as well, to tell his players like it is.

"I'd say, 'Guys, this is legal combat. It's a game that is violent, and you're going to have to compete against the other team physically, to show them that you're dominant over them. You can't go out there on the field thinking that you're something better, that you're not going to hit them hard.' You're going to have to be mentally strong so that you can dominate, then physically strong so that you can overwhelm them. That's the only way you can play.

"If players aren't technically sound or perfecting their techniques, they will probably get hurt," he says. "But, if they're concentrating on what they're supposed to do, they will not."

Richard wanted his players to know that they didn't have to be Neanderthals either. "They don't need to be cavemen about the game, to pound their chests when they hit someone. That's the macho part of the game, and they should be going out there with technique, with skill, and with verve to get the work done the right way."

He looks back on the old days. "You didn't see guys jumping up off the ground, pounding their chests, doing a war. That's because you were busy doing what you were supposed to do. It's your job as a team member. Today, some players seem more interested in themselves than in their teams. I couldn't be in the College Football Hall of Fame without my teammates. We wouldn't have been champions without our teammates. I would never be wearing a National Championship ring if it weren't for my teammates, and I've always let them know that."

Richard continues to think about how the game could be better played. He writes in a journal about how to teach kids to have more respect for the techniques and skills and less for the brutality.

He worries, too, about how to keep them away from drugs. Rich believes that steroid use actually contributes to player injuries. Steroids are used to alleviate pain and to make players' bodies bigger and stronger. But, they cause personality changes and internal injuries that affect other parts of their bodies. "It's a paradox in a way," he says, "These guys are just humongous, but at the end of practice, they're huffing and puffing, having difficulty breathing." He reiterates that they're still sweating long after practice is over and they're unable to move, to get off the bench and go home. "They're too juiced up."

When he was in junior high, Rich and his best friend Gil were lifting weights at the local YMCA when they were approached about taking "vitamins" to make them bigger. Neither had any idea what the young man was pushing. "My friend Gil said, 'Richie, he's talking about drugs, and I ain't messing with none of that stuff.' 'Me neither,'" Rich said.

He never used steroids but couldn't help but notice the rise in its use because of the differences in players. He told me that in the 1980s, players were bigger than those from the previous decade. By 1991, when he was coaching for the Bucs, he saw players become far more developed than they ought to have been. Linemen were getting huge, he told me. "Nowadays, young players don't use arm protection. They even roll up their sleeves to show off their guns [arms]."

Rich's old game tapes provide proof positive. In those, one can see that players were thinner and everyone wore arm pads to protect them from injury. None weighed 320 or more pounds, as some do now. Rich also noted that, in the last few years, he has read about young players weighing more than 350 pounds who have passed out, or even died, after practicing or playing. It's just too much weight to carry. Their hearts can't take it.

Besides, there's a whole lot more than size at play in football.

"Football is an art to me. There are a variety of techniques, much like martial arts," Richard explains. "You have so much to remember within a particular play and at a particular time. It may be only eight to ten seconds, but you have to remember everything because your feet and body have to be in a certain position, at a certain angle to accomplish what you want. It's just like when a tennis ball is coming at you. Your feet have to be just right in order for you to get the ball back in the line or wherever you want it to land. Linebackers are right up there where all the contact occurs. They need to know when to lower their heads and when not to. If someone is coming to block you, you can't put your head down. But, when you're getting ready to tackle, you should lower it. You need to remember that to avoid a neck injury. You just can't bury your head one minute and pop it out the next."

How you're coached makes a difference in how you play.

Rich's favorite coaches were his high school coaches, Frank Cicarell and Jack Von Bischoffhausen, otherwise known as Coach Von B. They were nice guys who didn't yell at the boys. "Coach Von B was a good guy. He cared about us," Rich says, tearing up. "He did everything in his power to help us be good people and good football players. If it wasn't for Coach Von B, I wouldn't have been a coach or even played football."

He hopes the game becomes less violent but has his doubts.

"It won't change. Look at what we're watching now with UFC," Rich says. "It's the ultimate fighting championship with bare hands and kicking, where they're drawing blood and using their whole bodies as weapons. They've gone completely violent, and some of that has, unfortunately, trickled down to high school and even little league."

Richard thinks it may get even worse. Until there are more deaths, more carnage—enough so that certain intellectuals can't stand it anymore, nothing will change. "Remember, they're making millions now," he says "So, there's little incentive to change."

Rich believes football has become more entertainment than anything. "And I feel partly responsible for the growth in Tampa. Because without the Bucs, where would we be? Would we have as much of a population as we do now if we didn't have professional entertainment from the Bucs or the Rays? Look at your major cities. The top four cities where everyone wants to live have professional teams."

On the plus side, football attracts people and business. It builds school loyalty, camaraderie, and pride. Fans and alumni are more willing to contribute to their colleges. It brings people together. Rich and Karen grew up in families that watched football. It was a large part of their lives, and remains so.

Fortunately, Karen had never had to see Rich being carted off the field on a stretcher in all the years that she watched him play. "It was like he was invincible," Karen says. "So, for me, I liked the sport. I'd get up there and yell with the fans. All our friends would come out to watch. But now, I see it as a brutal sport. It's like the gladiators yelling, 'kill, kill, kill.'"

Karen recalls seeing Richard's demeanor change because of football, though. There was a difference in him beginning in April and May that would last for several months. His personality changed. It took a few years to understand it, but it lasted more than a decade after he retired. "He was psyching himself up to play," she says.

Neither Richard nor Karen are sure they would want
their son to play now, after experiencing his football-related
health issues, but Marlon began playing high school football a
decade ago, and they were at his games then, cheering him
on. Knowing what they know now, they're sure they would
not want to see their young grandson play.

A casualty (he doesn't like "victim") of the violence in
football, Richard's long years of playing have taken a toll on
his health. In his second year playing football, back in junior
high, he sprained his knee. "But, with youth, you bounce back
fast. And, back then, they didn't take you to get x-rays so you
really didn't know what was happening."

When he was fifteen or sixteen and playing football in
the street, he broke his arm, shattering his elbow, which has a
tendency to lock up and continues to cause him pain. These
days, he said, most everything hurts—his shoulders, neck,
arms, his feet, his hands, and his back. He can't recall the
number of concussions he suffered, but guesses it was more
than a dozen, beginning in high school. "I remember being
taken out of games because I didn't know where I was."

Back then, he would be benched for one or two plays and
then be put back in again. "This was before we knew what
concussions could do, how long you should be out."

Even without a concussion, "Your equilibrium is totally
off—for awhile, anyway," he stated plaintively. "During the
first few plays of any game, you can't even see straight.
You're disoriented the minute the game starts. It's 'boom'
and you're running down the field and these guys are
waiting on you, cross-blocking you, or there are two or three
guys coming straight at you and it's 'bam' and you're
running at each other. It's part of the game to feel woozy, to
have to get acclimated to what's going to happen to you," he
says.

Richard is proud that he never missed a game because of injuries, but that didn't mean he wasn't hurt. "Yes, I tore my ankles up continuously, strained and hurt my back, had torn rib cartilage, concussions, lots of bumps, bruises, and soreness," he admits, "but it didn't stop me from playing. You shake it off, and you go to the sidelines and ask for smelling salts to clear your head. You just go on."

Why, one wonders? "You don't want to let your team down," Richard answers. "You want to do your best to compete. Besides, you don't want to lose your job. And, too, it's a macho thing. You ignore the pain. It's a violent game."

It's also the way the game is played.

"Nothing is like the physical contact that you have in football. I don't care what you train in — and I trained in Tae Kwon Do — your body is still going to go through some violence, even though you're not getting bullets shot at you as you would in war. Just the collision part of football, where you're running into each other for sixty minutes, is brutal." He asked me to imagine running full speed into a wall that's just ten feet away with a helmet and body gear on. It's going to hurt.

I can't help but ask if that scares him. "If you're afraid someone is going to hurt you — if you're scared to go out there to play, then you're in the wrong business. It's like being a soldier. If you're afraid to go to war, you shouldn't join the military."

Rich did get butterflies before a game, though. To offset them, he would go through a routine to relax his body. "I'd say to myself, 'Man, here we go again,' because I knew I had to get psyched up to go into battle. Football is physical. If you're scared, you'll make mistakes that might cost the team a touchdown."

Hiding pain isn't an easy thing with the whole world watching you.

But, ignore the pain he did...for years. After he stopped playing, Richard got to the point where he had trouble standing, sitting, lying down, or doing much of anything. All the years of absorbing blocks, tackling runners, and ignoring pain had stopped him.

He knew there was something wrong with his back and went to see the team doctor and other specialists more and more often. He thought the problem was muscular or arthritis, but beginning in 2000 or so he felt his spine shifting sideways, back and forth. "My spine would suddenly move and creak," he says.

He had trouble lifting anything over his head when demonstrating a play to his Wildcats team. He couldn't wear his bullet proof vest, although he was required to do so as a security resource officer. It caused too much pain.

An MRI finally painted the picture—Rich had nerve damage caused by crushed vertebrae, fractures, disc degeneration, and spondylosis.

Rich had an eight hour spinal surgery in 2007. Titanium rods and screws hold together three lumbar vertebrae. The fix helped but limited his mobility and flexibility. He still has sudden sharp pains and is unable to sit or stand for long periods of time.

Every doctor he has seen attributed his back problems to football. At this point, he is unable to work, although he would still love to coach or teach in some capacity.

Forced to seek assistance, Richard went to the NFL Retired Players Association for help. "But, a year after you've retired, the NFL doesn't want to have anything to do with you," he reluctantly states.

After a three-year-long legal battle, Richard Wood ended up receiving only eight months of disability benefits, each only $1800 before taxes. Rich was then forced to take early retirement at fifty-five or lose those benefits altogether. "They would not give me total and permanent disability."

As a pre-1993 football player, Rich could not get line-of-duty disability or other coverage that is available to post-1993 players. Yet, he belongs to the NFL Alumni Association. And what does he get with annual dues? "You get to play golf and get discount cards to rent cars at Avis, Hertz, and National," he said. Other than that, there are no benefits.

Talk about being a throwaway player.

Richard has no medical insurance although future surgeries loom. His feet, shoulders, hands, and one of his legs are all on his health agenda, as are two fingers that constantly numb up. He must walk slowly to avoid pain.

"I'm having trouble just moving the mouse on my computer. My shoulder will just fall out from the scarring that came from repeated torn ligaments." And with all those concussions, who knows whether he will fall victim to dementia or Alzheimer's disease some time down the line?

For the NFL to deny that concussions contribute to dementia is "just plain wrong," Richard says. They ought to recognize the fact that playing the game may cause harm later in life and provide former players with the help they need.

The NFL justifies its lack of support by saying that they're paying people good money to play. But the Jets paid Rich only $25,000 when he joined the club in 1975, and he grossed less than $800,000 for more than a decade of play. His income could certainly not justify the resulting medical expenses, pain, and suffering.

And the truth is that, until recently, players didn't know what the impacts of playing would have on the quality of their lives some twenty to thirty years after they left the field. No one told them playing could negatively affect the entire rest of their lives. Or that, for some, the game's violence could stimulate more violence.

"There's an old Chinese adage that from one comes two, and from two comes three, and so on," Richard says. "For some, then, violence begets more violence."

Fortunately, Richard wasn't one of those affected that way. Although often disappointed by the business of the game and hurting today from its after effects, he is thankful for football. It's how he met his wife, role models, and friends. It took him around the world and allowed him to meet people from many countries who love the game.

"Not for its brutality," he says wistfully, "but, for its beauty. You see guys jumping in mid-air and catching a ball while they're not even touching the ground. It's really artistic."

But Batman is the eternal optimist. "Things will get better," he says, rising ever so slowly to stand, simply ignoring the pain.

9

Injuries Are Real

In 1983, there was controversy surrounding violence and injuries in the National Football League. In a guest editorial for the *New York Times*, Michael Oriard wrote that violence and casualties were football's main attraction for fans and players. "Injuries are not aberrations in football, or even a regrettable by-product. They are essential to the game."

In fact, noted author James Michener pondered the football injury data of the 1970s in his book *Sports in America*. He posited that if physics classes were to annually kill twenty-eight students and injure 86% that, "...physics classes would be eliminated as a subject, and within a very short time, for such a cost would be deemed excessive...But there is no cry to end football, nor will there be, because every society decides what it is willing to pay for its entertainment."

I, too, was totally excited by a good hit, an outstanding block, a touchdown run. I was thrilled when the Buccaneers won a physical game. Our team was strong and fearless. Yes, I saw the injury report, but like most fans, I knew our players would be back in the game the following Sunday.

"This game is getting bigger, it's getting stronger and it's getting more dangerous. So that means what? More pain and more injuries," stated former Dallas Cowboys receiver Michael Irvin.

"We're coming to a point where our bodies just physically cannot take it anymore," Davin Joseph said in an interview with Joe Henderson of the *Tampa Tribune*. Joseph, a

6'3", 313 pound Tampa Bay All-Pro offensive lineman continued, "The equipment is better, but the explosion on contact is just so strong."

"You want to know how hard you're hit. If you are a running back, and you're hit full speed, he can literally knock the feces out of your bowels. You lose all feeling in your limbs. That's how hard they hit in the NFL," says Merrill Hoge, a former Steelers and Bears running back who left the game in 1985 due to serious concussions suffered on the field.

Howard News Service's Thomas Hargrove writes about how devastating injuries are a result of two factors: body mass and physics. In the 1980's it was rare for a player to weigh 300 pounds. William "Refrigerator" Perry who played for the Bears got more press attention for his size (370 pounds) than his play on the field. He scored a touchdown in Super Bowl XX in 1986. That fact is usually lost. Perry was a freak in the National Football League at that time. Now his size approaches the norm for some positions. In the summer of 2005, more than five hundred training camp attendees weighed 300 pounds or more.

Rob Zatechka, former NFL player and currently an anesthesiologist, raises an interesting point about fitness with a Body Mass Index (BMI) that categorized him as obese during his playing days, yet he maintained a level of twelve percent body fat.

The NFL has promoted this idea that lean body mass is safe mass. The weight on the muscles and ligaments, however, remains the same. The stress on the cardiovascular system remains unchanged. Weight is weight. Stop a minute and consider where this weight originates. What substance builds lean muscle mass?

Anabolic steroids.

This increase in weight coincides with the introduction of performance enhancing substances into the National Football League.

This bulk harms the players' own bodies putting them at greater risks for heart attacks, strokes, and diabetes as well as disintegrating joints and ligament damage. It also leads to substantial force upon collision with another player on the field.

Brushing up on my physics by reading Tim Gray's book *Football Physics: the Science of the Game*, I was reminded of Newton's third law: Conservation of Momentum. This basically translates to the fact that whenever two players collide, no matter size differences or how fast each is traveling, they always exert the same amount of force on each other. The impact is the same for each player, however, in opposite directions. For example, if a player of 245 pounds tackles a player of 185, they both sustain an impact of 1150 pounds of force. Multiply this play by the number of tackles in a game, and you begin to understand why linemen last an average of 2.6 years in the National Football League.

While the players' joints are an obvious target of abusive practices, the heart is also at risk. In March of 2008, researchers at Mayo Clinic announced the findings of a study that looked at "the cardiovascular health of 233 retired NFL players, aged 35-65. They did this by measuring the internal diameter of the carotid (neck) artery and by assessing levels of plaque deposits that can block blood flow. The researchers found that 82 percent of the retired players under the age 50 had abnormal narrowing and blockage in their arteries greater than the 75th percentile of the general population."

Retirement brings a harsh reality to players. Upon initially accepting their signing bonuses, few players factor in the data that insurance only covers them for five years after playing. No insurance carrier wants to enroll a former NFL player. A Scripps Howard News Service study reported that football players were twice as likely to die before the age of fifty as Major League Baseball players. Of the players to die before fifty, many of those suffered from obesity or side effects of obesity.

From what I have witnessed, most players have physical injuries that do not end within five years. These injuries are cumulative both on bodies and brains. Arthritis keeps progressing with time.

In December 2009, Conrad Dobler began promoting his autobiography *Pride and Perseverance*. A three time Pro Bowl guard in the1970s with a reputation for being a hard-partying, hard-living player, Dobler had been off the radar screen for almost thirty years.

Playing ten years in the NFL, where the average playing time for his position is less than three years, took its toll on Dobler's knees. With the help of painkillers, he endures the aftermath of thirty-two knee surgeries and eight knee replacements. He currently battles a persistent staph infection lodged in the knee and fights the idea of amputation.

Michael O'Keeffe wrote an article in the *New York Daily News* on Conrad, and he had this to say about the time when Conrad first started having knee problems after retirement. Conrad had an attorney "call the NFL Players' Association to get some information about applying for disability. He was put on hold and transferred to twelve different people. He was on the phone for thirty-five minutes and never actually talked to anybody. He hung up and told me, 'They aren't going to do anything for you, Conrad.' That gave me a glimpse of what was to come."

While it is reasonable to assume a former player in his late fifties would suffer arthritis from football injuries, one does not expect a retiree of thirty-six to be in a similar situation. In 2007, Michael McCrary, a former lineman for the Ravens, discussed his retirement reality with John Eisenberg of the *Baltimore Sun*.

As a Raven, McCrary traveled to the Pro Bowl twice and won a Super Bowl ring. At 240 pounds, he was small to be playing on the line where these days the average weight is over 300 pounds. McCrary compensated with strength and drive and destroyed his knees in the process. When the Ravens signed him to a five year contract extension in 1999, he had already undergone four knee surgeries.

In the middle of the 2001 season, McCrary's mother intervened.

Sandy McCrary said, "I don't think Michael ever really understood the full ramifications of some of what was going on. He always had been able, through his strong work ethic, to make things better, so he was convinced if he rehabilitated hard and did all he was told, this situation would get better. He never understood that after all the chop blocks and people taking him out, his condition was so bad that the all the rehab in the world was not going to help him. That was so contrary to his way of thinking.

"It clicked for him when I said to seek an opinion from non-NFL doctors, and he heard he had the knees of a 70-year old. And that they were only going to get worse.

Months before he reached thirty, McCrary was a Super Bowl winner. That January day in 2001, he received a cortisone injection. As he explained to Eisenberg, "It was the biggest game of my life." And McCrary was in pain.

Later that year he was out of football. His knees could not continue.

His knees can barely support his weight. In 2007, he confessed to the *Baltimore Sun* reporter, "I've been on Percocet, Percodan, OxyCotin, Oxycodone, and three different psychiatric medicines. I had a fentanyl patch; that's like heroin. I 'm on methadone now."

According to an article written by Carl Prine, their union claims that nearly half of all NFL players depart the game due to injuries that preclude further play. Approximately a quarter of these athletes have degenerative bone/joint conditions or experience chronic traumatic encephalopathy from repeated concussions.

Currently, only two percent of retired players receive any type of NFL disability benefit, partial or permanent.

Because NFL contracts are basically a series of one-year agreements, players stay on the field as long as possible. Ignoring injuries and the concomitant pain, they take the field to secure the incentives which are built into their contracts.

With the exception of a few key players, no contract is guaranteed. If the player is injured for the season and not on the field, there is no paycheck on Monday. Additionally, most signing bonuses are back-end loaded. According to team management, this is done in order to relieve the salary cap. Don't believe it. If a player is injured permanently, the remaining money in the bonus is gone.

Andrew Zimbalist, economics professor at Smith College, claims that the average salary in the NFL was around $1.3 million in 2006. Surprised? Don't be. Only the sensational salaries get publicized. Yes, $1.3 million per year is a fortune, but when you realize the average football career lasts less than three years, it becomes problematic. Additionally, these players are in the upper tax bracket forcing them to pay fifty-five percent of their salary to the IRS.

Since over half the players leave the league due to debilitating injuries, it is difficult to find meaningful employment post-NFL. It is difficult to stand or sit or walk with crippling joint pain. It is difficult to reason if you've been concussed. Applying for benefits seems the appropriate thing to do. However, players must swallow their pride to do so.

The players union's director of benefits states that there are five hundred annual claims for disability payments that come from football injuries, but there's not enough money to pay them. Carl Prine, in his *Tribune Review* article, mirrored my thoughts when he wrote, "They're truly disposable parts, which is something they've been for a long time in terms of the owners — and now the fans."

The director of benefits also points out that the union annually funds more than $10.5 million for retired players' medical bills. However, most players never amass enough money during their careers to pay the out-of-pocket costs for long term conditions such as arthritis or cardiovascular disease. After studying a self-funding insurance program, the union deemed it too expensive to be feasible.

Mike Ditka, a Hall of Fame Coach and player for the Chicago Bears, argues that older players who built the league should be treated with more respect. "Don't make proud men beg." In response to what Ditka views as injustices to former players, he formed Gridiron Greats, an organization that provides emergency funds to players in need.

One of the stumbling blocks to disabled players accessing benefits through their union is the reluctance of current players to fund the program. Current players want the union to represent their interests both with management and in merchandizing agreements. They see retired players as an economic drag. They never consider the fact that they, too, will one day be retired with a fifty percent chance of having a lasting disability.

Unfortunately, no retired players sit as voting trustees on the NFLPA board. After paying dues during and after their careers, they are denied representation in assessing applications for disability payments. These decisions are solely in the hands of current players, and they have no interest in paying out more money for disabled players' benefits.

Miki Yaras-Davis, NFLPA's director of benefits has a striking description. She calls it the "underbelly of the sport" — an unseen line of broken older, thrown away players struggling to pay their medical bills.

However, as Scot Brantley has said many times, "When you are retired, it's like you are wiped off the face of the earth There is a lot of need out there. I'd say eighty percent of the guys who played need some kind of help, but it's hard to get. There's something wrong with the system."

10

Nathan Fisher: the Future of Football

Like many people, I hate shots. Some friends would say I border on being phobic. I have tried to develop tactics to make the situation more tolerable. My latest attempt went rather well. I decided to get to know my torturer, turn her into an ally, and pray for the best. So you don't think I am a total wuss, these shots have to be given very slowly over several minutes AND they really sting. They hurt actually.

The nurse enters the cubicle and I begin talking — perhaps too quickly? She has a son, Nathan, who is nine years old. He plays football on a local league. I have a grandson who is nine and plays football in another state. Max wants to play football at the University of Florida. Nathan wants to be a Gator as well. Max made the All-Star team his first year of play. Nathan was a standout player for the last two years.

As I left the office, we exchanged children's names and promised to meet in the stands when her son and my grandson were teammates in Gainesville, Florida. The shot went well, but our conversation stayed with me. Her parting statement to me was that when Nathan "made it big," she'd get a new house and retire.

I hope Nathan Fisher "makes it big," but the odds are against him. He lives in a very small Florida town of less than five thousand people with one high school. The University of Florida is a two hour drive, a short distance geographically, but a long road for an aspiring athlete. It is becoming increasingly difficult to achieve admission to UF. Everyone wants to attend the winning school: the 2008 National Football Champions. The University of Florida wins national titles regularly, so only the most talented players become Gators.

This is the first hurdle for Nathan in his quest to "make it big." Playing high school football in a small town will lessen his chances of being scouted by universities. His coach will have to promote him as a prospect by sending DVD's of his performances in local games and following up with calls to the athletic director. Additionally, Nathan will have to maintain high grades and have good off-field conduct. No coach can offer scholarships to students with pre-existing problems these days.

Unfortunately, playing prep football is time consuming. From elementary school level through high school, the player exists in an excited state of concentrating on football to the detriment of academic performance. There are daily practices and training exercises that leave the students too fatigued to fully devote the time necessary to successfully comprehend class work or homework.

To complicate matters, football is no longer seasonal. There are weight and strength programs year-round for the committed athlete. There is competition to make the roster year after year. There is no time off.

The players at every school level form a special clique. They become a brotherhood- a true team. It's addicting to be wanted and praised for one's athletic prowess. Unfortunately, intellectuals are rarely wanted and/or praised for their achievements at this level. Hence, it is even easier for the football player to ignore academics. This is a downfall for those who hope to play on a top university team. It's truly the first challenge of a young player.

Many high profile football universities understand their athletes' dilemma. Most provide tutoring and academic supports for athletic teams who travel to games or meets. Some go so far as to recommend "easy A" courses. However, more than a few universities offer their athletes the ultimate gift: someone to give you the answers to an online test and/or write your papers for you.

Florida State Penalized in Academic Fraud Case
New York Times   (page B-9)
Written by: Lynn Zinser
March 7, 2008

The N.C.A.A. ruled that Florida State University (FSU) was guilty of major violations in a widespread academic fraud case uncovered in 2007. On March 6, 2009, the N.C.A.A. announced that it would strip scholarships from 10 Seminole teams and force them to vacate all of the victories in 2006 and 2007 in which the implicated students participated. In addition, the (university) was placed on probation for four years."

The N.C.A.A. committee determined that beginning in 2006 several academic personnel wrote papers and took tests fir athletes enrolled in a music class.

This is but one example, and one made public because Florida State University is known as a football powerhouse. Unfortunately for the athletes involved, their education is not of primary importance. Their ability to thrill the donors and alum with their winning record is their value to the university.

Many athletes fail to leave college with a degree. If they aren't picked up by a professional sports team, they have few marketable skills with which to support themselves.

Alternatively, the athlete may graduate with a degree made up of courses that he did not attend. His homework was done for him, reports were written, and tests taken by academic support staff. I witnessed this fallout far too often at the Buccaneers. Time and time again, players were unable to read their contracts or understand their playbooks. BUT they were *college graduates*!

Sons like Nathan have familial and economic pressure to perform. There are maternal expectations that nine year old Nathan will one day provide. This is his family's way out of a small apartment in a rural town. Of course, he will "make it big;" he has to for his family's financial survival.

This is the pressure that will lead Nathan to take extreme means to be competitive. He will readily ingest anything that promises a quicker, stronger body. He, like many others, is not concerned with long-term side effects. He needs to make the team and retain his position.

And believe me, Nathan will have plenty of company. It is well known by now that the dependence on performance enhancing substances is widespread among aspiring athletes of all ages, along with their professional counterparts.

The International Olympic Committee and the National Collegiate Athletic Association have prohibited anabolic steroids and ephedrine for use in competition. Blood transfusions are also forbidden. However, growth hormones are a factor now. As ex-Raider Howie Long stated, "It's undetectable. It's the ultimate football drug."

A Stanford University study wrote that, "Human growth hormone (hGH) is produced naturally in the body, regulating height and muscle and organ growth. A synthetic version is approved by the U.S. Food and Drug Administration for children with growth disorders (e.g., Turner Syndrome) and AIDS patients who suffer dangerous weight loss."

So now we have the key. Since the human growth hormone is produced naturally within the athlete's body, how can it be detected? Added to this is the fact that the synthetic hormone has an incredibly short half-life (the amount of time it stays in the body). It can be detected through elaborate and expensive measures, but only at the time of peak performance or within twenty-four to thirty-six hours from the last administration of the hormone.

The National Football League as well as the International Olympic Committee banned athletes' use of human growth hormone. Baseball similarly banned the substance. In January 2007, the FDA emphasized that prescribing or distributing human growth hormone for non-medical reasons was illegal.

Still athletes use the hormone. Why? Because it works. In the few studies conducted, human growth hormone was shown to increase lean muscle mass.

Interestingly these scientific studies never tested the high doses of human growth hormone that athletes routinely use. The scientific thought is that it could be dangerous to the subjects, and the hormones required would be prohibitively expensive.

Additionally, athletes have become their own pharmacists. They combine the anabolic effects of steroids with the anabolic effects of human growth hormone which also has the added benefit of being able to hide within the body. One could call this the perfect medical storm or the path to fame and glory in the National Football League. Dexter Manly, former Buccaneer and ex-Redskins lineman, summed it up when he said, "Everything is so competitive. It's like when people want to speed on the highway, so they buy radar detectors…People on steroids use these growth hormones to outdo the cops."

When the scientists have cracked the code to detect the human growth hormone, there will be other ergogenics to replace them. Recombinant human growth hormone is now being used for anabolic purposes.

Joining rhGH is insulin-like growth factor-I (IGF-I), as well as insulin, which is also being used "off label" by amateur and professional athletes in their quest to get bigger, stronger and faster.

Nathan will also face an onslaught of designer drugs tailored to meet the separate needs of each athlete. Now that genes have been mapped, expect genetic engineering and manipulation to enhance athletic prowess. How will the world Anti-Doping Agency (WADA) keep pace?

What will happen to Nathan's body and mind as he tries to "make it big"? Will he suffer cardiovascular disease from anabolic drug use or depression and psychosis from concussions? Will he beat the odds and buy his mother a house on his NFL paycheck? OR will Nathan Fisher question the ethos of a society that sacrifices its young athletes' health for the pleasure of the fans and then throws them away when they're done?

11

Student Athletes

Parent education is a top priority in youth sports. Often times, the team coach in community leagues is a father or uncle; the same with the trainer. They have no special training but have the willingness to volunteer their precious time to the team. Therefore, it is imperative that parents be aware of safety issues and knowledgeable in reducing and preventing injuries.

I strongly suggest that parents disapprove of the use of performance enhancing substances and emphasize to their children the importance of playing with their natural talents. Parents need to understand the long-term consequences of steroid use and the use of human growth hormones. Many times, I have listened to mothers trying to justify why they requested growth hormones from their child's pediatrician. In my world, there simply is no case for these drugs in the world of competitive sports. As a society, we need to learn to play with our natural bodies; not those that are pumped up to super-human proportions.

I interviewed William G. Carson, M.D., a physician specializing in sports medicine. From his years of experience in treating student athletes, he had the following recommendations for parents, athletes, and coaches concerning healthy competition:

> I think that being a member of a sports team, at any level, under the right circumstances and coach supervision, has many benefits for any child:

understanding team work, building confidence and self-esteem, beginning to understand that every sports season will have its ups and downs and you will not win every game, learning to accept defeat gracefully and learn from it. It is only from some of our failures that we really grow and appreciate those times when things go our way and we win. In short, I feel that being on some type of sports team at a young age has more advantages than the disadvantage that an injury may occur.

The best sport for a child is one he or she will enjoy and one that has adult supervision by trained individuals. There are those classic Little League parents who sit in the stands at the games and yell and scream at not only the coach but at their own child. This is a very unhealthy environment for children and will probably deter them from future sports endeavors. The situation is even magnified when young kids play "pee wee" football because the coaches can be very aggressive and teach the kids to hit each other and "be tough". Unfortunately, outside of a school sport, most coaches are parent-volunteers and have very little training in sports injuries. I feel that at a minimum they should all be trained in basic first aid, injury recognition and CPR. However, it is really pot luck as to what kind of coach will show up.

Christopher Nowinski, Co-Director of the Center for the Study for Traumatic Encephalopathy at the Boston University School of Medicine and the President and CEO of the Sports Legacy Institute, presented the data on concussions this way before the Congressional committee:

I hope we can recast this issue as a public health crisis. We must remember that 95% of football players are under the age of 18 and under the age of consent. So the idea that "we know what we are getting into" is erroneous.

• We must also remember that this affects millions of young boys. In fact, one in eight high school boys play football in America, and millions more participate at the junior high and elementary levels.

• We must remember that the young, developing brain is more sensitive to trauma.

• We must remember that younger players have weaker necks than adults, making head trauma more damaging to the brain. In fact, a recent study out of the University of Illinois actually found high school players take greater forces to the brain than college players.

• We must remember that most concussions, perhaps as many as 90%, go undiagnosed.

• We must remember that that nearly half of players, even when diagnosed, return to play too soon, before their brains have had the chance to recover physiologically.

• And we must remember that most children don't have access to medical care or oversight at football practices or games. Less than half of high schools have athletic trainers.

Merrill Hoge played for the Pittsburgh Steelers and the Chicago Bears from 1987 until 1994, when he retired due to a preponderance of head injuries. Subsequently, he became a youth football coach. When he testified before the House

Judiciary Committee at which I was present, he told a story I could not get out of my head. Unfortunately, it is a story that could be told in every city every day.

"I had a young kid named Griffin, who got up from a collision and was a little woozy. He had sustained some kind of head trauma. As I pulled him to the side, ironically, his older brother, Jake, helps coach. He is twenty-five years old. Now, Jake obviously knows Griffin much better than I, although I know Griffin very well. I wanted to address a lot of cognitive things that I am aware of now—from retrograde to anterograde, to his name, to what play we just ran, to find out where his senses were, looking at his pupils—some of the things I know. Then I asked Jake to sit and talk to him and make sure that he didn't elevate from sickness to dizziness.

"Well, after five minutes, Jake ran up to me and said, 'Grif is ready to go back in.' And I'm like. 'No. Grif is done playing.' I just wanted to make sure that the symptoms didn't elevate so that we could get him to the hospital. Then after the game, I could talk to his parents about monitoring him and taking him to the doctor if necessary.

"The caution and concern I have is that Jake could very easily be a head coach in our youth program, and he was willing to put his own brother back on the football field, purely out of ignorance."

Starting with the Pee Wee players, coaching is important. It is more important at this stage than at any other. If one doesn't learn the correct way to tackle, run or throw at age seven, poor habits will haunt the player as he grows.

If a coach teaches the player correctly, he builds the foundation of a good football player. Otherwise, the results can be disastrous. What if Jake was the primary coach and Griffin went back into the game and suffered a second concussion? What does the coach teach the other players on the team, and what does he teach the parents. This is youth football—Pee Wee ball—not the National Football League. The NFL is clear. Griffin would not have been allowed back in the game.

As I speak to retired players across the country, they invariably tell me their first concussion was as a young player in a youth league. They cannot even tally for me the number of times they were "dinged." They were taught, however, to get up and get back in the game. That macho football mantra is ingrained from early on in their football lives. No one wants a cry-baby on the team.

Children get to the point that it is a matter of honor not to tell your coach or your mother that you suffered a head injury. This behavior needs to halt immediately. These young boys will be thrown to the curb very quickly if they can't remember which way to run or whom to block. They will not be invited to play on the team the following year. Before their career has begun, it will be over. They will have feelings of insecurity, and they might possibly have residual brain damage.

No one but you and your son really cares whether or not he plays the following year unless he has an arm like Brett Farve. Otherwise, he'll be forgotten. There will be no team celebrations or dinners with other players. He will be an outcast because he is no longer on the team. His ego will take a hit as will his popularity at school and in the neighborhood.

Players I speak with on this topic always counsel that students need to rely on good grades for college, not football or sport scholarships. The reason is simple: If you are injured, there is no athletic scholarship.

How many parents and students count on getting an athletic scholarship? Too many. I hear it in the stands all the time. In any sport, the talk is of the college scholarship. High school coaches push this idea to get the best performance from their players. Parents push their children so that they can save the tuition dollars. In all of this pressure, the child tries too hard, perhaps takes a few steroids, to boost his performance and then is injured.

Parents need to see college scholarships realistically, and they need to access their child's talents realistically. And as retired players suggest, they need to stay in school and plan for a career outside of sports. Very few students become college athletes, and even fewer become professional athletes. Parents need to stress this fact to their children.

12

My Journey Continues

While I was an administrator for the Tampa Bay Buccaneers, I saw things that I questioned. Of course, being a female in a man's world, I did not voice my concerns. I figured it was better to keep my own counsel and see what transpired. I assumed the coaches and trainers and the doctors knew more than I could ever imagine. Still, visions and questions clouded my thoughts. Common sense told me that things didn't make sense. But who would have listened to me in the late 80s? I had a doctorate from Columbia University in mental retardation; I had no football experience.

A few years ago, I read an article about Richard Wood, a former Buccaneer linebacker where he discussed his constant pain from arthritis and multiple surgeries due to injuries suffered while playing football. He also stated that he was nearing bankruptcy.

I flew to Tampa and began tracking former players. I was shocked by what I heard and saw. These men were and are suffering. Some have no short term memory, some can only stand for a few minutes due to back pain, some have extreme migraine headaches, some are addicted to pain medication, and many players have lost major cognitive function. One had committed suicide.

As I mourned what I experienced, I decided something needed to be done immediately to stop the carnage of these young men on the field. I began writing. I had to find a way to share my knowledge.

The woman in the front office would be silent no more.

I researched football related injuries for two years. I looked at football players' weights through multi-year studies. This led me to performance enhancing substances and the physics of two players driving into one another. Of course, this made me question the impact on the brain and early onset dementia and Chronic Traumatic Encephalopathy (CTE). This morphed into research on concussion-induced depression and the deaths of players at their own hands.

Throughout all of this research was the undercurrent of a society that is fixated on violence and the overarching question of why we allow violence to persist on and off the field. What draws spectators to acts of violence? Why are players held to a different standard of leniency as the law is concerned?

I became obsessed. I sought out like-minded people to discuss my findings. I argued with those opposed to my ideas. I wanted to make certain I was not missing anything. Their arguments solidified my thinking. My former players became my sounding board. With their encouragement and enthusiasm, I pressed for change.

With the help of friends, I was invited to address the House Judiciary Committee on "Legal Issues Relating to Football Head Injuries" convened on October 28, 2009. As I got ready to testify, I spoke with one of my former players. He reminded me of what he called me, "A rebel, but a rebel with a cause. Gay, make them hear that we are hurt. Make them hear that we cannot fill out all of their forms. We can't do it. Our mental capacity isn't there to answer the questions on the phone and fill out the forms. They are missing those of us who are severely disabled."

Scot Brantley was my coach; his was the pep talk I needed. I strode into the hearing representing my players and advocating reform. I was seated in front of the committee at a table with Roger Goodell, the commissioner of the National Football League, and DeMaurice Smith, the players' union executive director, along with several male doctors representing various entities. Once again, I was the lone woman in the NFL world. However, this time I spoke the truth as I experienced it. I was silent no longer.

I spoke with the passion that had been building for years. I spoke for players who had no voice. I felt total freedom in that room. I had nothing to lose. No one could censor me. The truth flew from my lips.

I spoke of the injustices done to the players who were put back on the field with injuries. Players forced themselves to play with concussions. They knew their back-up wanted on the field. They had to hold onto their jobs. I described the players who were injected with pain killers in the locker rooms so they could continue after half time.

These players, these men, had been thrown away after their years of gripping our hearts with their plays. What remained were the broken bodies and lost souls of the men who have permanently left the locker room. This is what remains after the cheering subsides. This is what the National Football League does not want you to see.

I decided I could no longer stand by and do nothing. As damaging as steroids are, I came to understand this devastating nemesis that affected athletes, which led to the birth of The Gay Culverhouse Players' Outreach Program, Inc.

In March 2010, I hosted a meeting of retired players in Tampa to explain my players' outreach program. Fifty players attended. One after another they shuffled in, the victims of deteriorating joints, spinal fusions, and dementia.

Greg Roberts, an Outland Trophy winner, still has that great smile, but he is suffering horrible pain from arthritis.

John Reaves is coping the best he can, but he doesn't realize he keeps repeating the same words. We are respectful. Everyone is suffering.

Like many of you, I have watched older relatives start to repeat themselves. We patiently listen to the same story five times in an hour. We understand this is part of their aging process. The doctors tell us they are suffering the onset of senile dementia or Alzheimer's disease. Although we may be distressed, we understand.

Upon returning to the Tampa area after fifteen years, I met players whom I hardly recognized. When I looked closely I could see that smile I remembered, and I could hear that deep voice from the past. But without an introduction, I'd never have recognized my former players.

Scot Brantley was an exception. He was still the strapping physical essence of a linebacker. I was relieved until he spoke. Recently he had lost his position at a local sports radio station. While on the air he suffered a stroke and couldn't speak. He didn't know where he was. Months later, Scot repeats himself and looses his thoughts in the middle of a sentence. He writes notes in the palm of his hand to remember what he needs.

During his football career, Scot sustained multiple concussions. He is now moving to be closer to his family who can help him with his heart problems and the fact that he is now blind in one eye. If that weren't enough, my friend is concussed. He and I know he is losing cognitive function because his brain is compromised from his hard hitting playing days.

Before too long, Scot won't recognize me. I'll always picture him in his glory days: the days of dignity when he realized he was losing his mind and asked how he could help other players.

We hired Scot as a spokesman for The Gay Culverhouse Players' Outreach Program, Inc. because he knew the players, and they respected him league wide. He did public service announcements for us and spoke to player groups about the importance of seeking benefits from the NFL to which the former players were entitled. Unfortunately, players don't know they are entitled to a wide range of benefits from playing in the league, and Scot helped us spread that word in the initial phases of our program.

He was also my inside man who helped me understand what happens to retired players — how they disappear, and the sad state of their finances. He coached me well and prepared me for my presentation to Congress. There were things that needed to be said, and he made certain I heard them.

When I spoke before Congress, it was for Scot and hundreds of other former players. Scot was also very instrumental in helping our fledgling organization meet players of other alumni groups. He introduced us to the men we needed to know in order to spread the word around the NFL cities. Scot's help was invaluable. When we needed him the most, he was there for us.

Fortunately, through the help of Scot, Batman, and other players, we have been able to reach a great number of men who need services that are provided by the NFL. The major problem is getting that information to the players. There is a gap between what the league offers in terms of benefits and the knowledge of how to access those benefits. That is where our outreach comes in to play. We bridge that gap. We hold meetings around the country and help players get the evaluations they need to apply for services provided by the NFL.

Sadly, this leads to some alarming encounters. One player came to me and said, "Gay, I'm thirty-nine, and I can't remember anything. Can you help me? It's not right. I'm only thirty-nine. What's happening to me?"

I introduced him to a doctor that very night. (At most meetings we have a neurologist present with us.) Unfortunately, and not unusually, he failed to appear for his appointment the following week. We tried to track him down, but his phone was disconnected. His wife hadn't heard from him. He was scared and on the run. And that's the problem—many players don't want to face what lies ahead for them.

When your future consists of knowing that you'll lose your memory and your ability to know where you are, or how to dress yourself, it's natural to want to run from that reality. We have more than a few players make appointments never to show up for them. They do not want the truth. I'm not certain I'd want it either.

This fact is what leads many players to use drugs. It is an escape. They aren't addicts, they're just men trying to forget or cope with their impending doom. I have gotten to the point where I assume players are using some drug just to get through the day. I understand it. Their confusion is so great that it's one thing they have control over. Getting high to escape the confusion seems a reasonable reaction.

We had an orthopedist call one day and ask if we could see a patient of his. He was a former Buccaneer and was being seen for an arthritic knee. My reply was simple and immediate. "Of course, we'll call him today."

Well, we did. He had been in Tampa a few weeks and had already been picked up for drugs several times. Before he left for Florida, he had been arrested approximately five times in Alabama for drug possession. He needed help. As a former linebacker, football had taken its toll on him. Although he hadn't played in the NFL for a long time, he had been a huge college standout known for his rough play. His ex-wife was helping him get treatment for his knees and looking to us to help get his NFL benefits. She was standing by him knowing that without her help, he would be homeless.

Being in this business, I often think of that county western song "Mamas, Don't Let Your Babies Grow-up to be Cowboys," only I substitute "football players." This is a dangerous sport, and it takes its toll.

I remember waiting for an appointment in Starbucks. A hunched over grey haired man entered, but I didn't pay any attention and only looked up briefly before returning to my newspaper. The old man slowly made his way over to my table. "Gay?" There he was—Richard Wood, the legendary "Batman" of the Buccaneers' 1979 division-winning team. The man I stared at looked like he'd barely survived a train wreck.

The reporter with me had several questions, but I could barely speak. I was in shock. Football had done its damage to my son's favorite player. I didn't tell my son about the meeting. I couldn't.

Another prime example of being beaten up, used up, and thrown away is Jerry Eckwood. Jerry Eckwood (#88) played for the Buccaneers from 1979, when he was drafted in the third round (ahead of Joe Montana), until he left the team in 1981. In his three year career, Eckwood rushed five hundred fifteen times for 1845 yards and six touchdowns, and was a starter in thirty of forty-seven games. He caught ninety-five passes for nine hundred fifty-six yards and one touchdown. He was a key member of the first playoff appearance in 1979. Doug Williams was his quarterback, and John McKay was his coach.

In January 2009, I reviewed former Buccaneer players who had played from 1976-1994. Tom McHale was dead, a victim of CTE. I was working against time before I lost another player. I reached out to former players who were with the Bucs in the early years. My question? Who did they think might be in need?

One name surfaced repeatedly: Jerry Eckwood. "He's bad, Gay, really bad off."

From the stands, I witnessed Jerry heading to the opposing team's bench when our defense took the field. I watched as our players led him to our huddle as he stumbled in mid-field. These are the actions of a confused player, one who is disoriented. In hindsight, Eckwood was obviously suffering the effects of concussions.

Over thirty years later, players are coming to me with reports of Jerry's disorientation after practices at One Buccaneer Place. Often times, Jerry would sit in the locker room long after practice ended. When asked why, he replied, "Man, I don't know where home is." His teammate stepped in and drove him home, another drove his car for him.

Many saw Jerry's confusion but no one in the 70s knew how to handle it. Concussion data was non-existent. More than a few players were getting their "bells rung" or suffering "dings" to their heads. This was part of the game; it was accepted behavior. No one saw it as a problem.

As Jerry more frequently ran the wrong pattern, the quarterback was throwing into the arms of the opposition. Running assignments were scrambled; Jerry was never where he was expected to be. The fans decided that the quarterback was blind or his throwing arm was malfunctioning. The coaches and players knew the truth. They alone knew what plays had been called. The "BOO's" went to the quarterback, which was an unfounded derision.

Eckwood became a liability. With no short term memory and relying solely on teammates to steer him around the field, his services to the team were no longer needed.

In January 2009, I asked former Bucs who played with Jerry to help me find him. Batman Wood had heard from him several months ago. Others had word that he was in Little Rock,

Arkansas, his hometown. All said that they heard he wasn't doing well.

We obtained his girlfriend's cell phone number in Little Rock. Unfortunately, that number was no longer in use. Through diligent work, a friend of mine found Eckwood's nephew who was playing college ball. His coach was contacted. Being extremely helpful, he gave us Jerry's daughter's contact information.

In a fortunate coincidence, Jerry was living in a neighboring town and had a working cell phone. By this point, over nine months had passed. I thought our journey was almost complete. I was terribly mistaken.

Finding Jerry turned out to be the easy part. I asked Mitchell Welch to continue the work he had begun. He had done such a great job locating Jerry, so I thought one more favor would be a piece of cake. I asked him to get the NFL benefits paperwork to Jerry and walk him through the process to obtain his NFL disability benefits.

Mitchell spoke with Jerry's daughter. She would oversee the completion of the forms and get Jerry to the doctor for an evaluation. Weeks passed. Mitchell tried to contact Jerry. On the days they spoke, Mitchell was asked again who he was and what he wanted. Eckwood had no memory of previous calls. It was like the movie, *Groundhog Day*, and the pattern kept repeating. Jerry's daughter was finding it difficult to help her father.

Mitchell was facing disappointment as well. He thought Jerry would be thrilled to have the funds to which he is entitled. Jerry asked repeatedly if he could get money to pay off his credit card debt. Mitchell again explained the NFL benefits were for injuries suffered during his NFL career.

His daughter lost interest. It became more and more difficult to reach Jerry. If Mitchell spoke with him in the afternoon, he was incoherent; before noon, he had no memory of the call. He began to think Jerry had no interest in our help and surmised that he was more interested in getting high.

I explained that drinking to dull the physical pain and a confused mind was normal behavior for a concussed player. I reminded Mitchell of Jerry's confusion on the field during game days. This was a logical progression in a man who was suffering dementia at an early age. If Jerry was eighty years old, this behavior could be considered expected and accepted.

The problem is one does not understand how a vital fifty-four year old former athlete can deteriorate to such an extensive degree. Jerry, along with many retired players, has lost his ability to do what is in his best interest. If you can't find your way home in your twenties, you can't begin to understand the complexities of the NFL benefits in your fifties.

The public expects injuries on game day like broken bones, strained groins, and colliding heads. However, since most players return to play within at least a few games, it never crosses our mind that thirty years later the effects of those incidences manifest in significant ways. Knees and hips need to be replaced, and back surgery is required. Pills are needed to quiet the constant pain. The brain is being destroyed by the toxin Tau. Of all the injuries, the concussions are the most devastating. With a rapidly deteriorating brain, dementia and depression are a surety.

Jerry Eckwood does not understand what is happening. It's useless to try to explain the complexities of Chronic Traumatic Encephalopathy to him. He is most likely entitled to benefits under the 88 Plan. Through our foundation, we have paid for Mitchell to visit Jerry in Tennessee many times. We shall not leave him in his time of distress. Mitchell has taken Jerry to several doctors at Vanderbilt Medical Center.

He has been evaluated by the doctors and they determined he has dementia. He has, with our foundation's help, applied for the 88 Plan. We are waiting now for the NFL to determine his eligibility. We hope that Jerry will be able to live in an assisted living facility. We want him to have daily activities to look forward to and to have people to share his meals with and talk with and share his day. Jerry has been alone far too long.

A funny thing happened on this road. Jerry, who was originally suspicious and downcast, now considers Mitchell to be his best friend. They talk every day by phone. With his permission, Jerry has been featured in the *New York Times*, the *Tampa Tribune*, the *Sarasota Herald* and ESPN. He no longer feels forgotten. He is upbeat and happy to have new friends that remember him.

Football is endemic to our culture. Football programs raise money for universities. Professional teams enhance the financial status of NFL cities. Three hours of televised play highlighting a city is a Chamber of Commerce's dream. Florists, caterers, restaurants, taxi companies, cleaners, and all forms of businesses benefit from football in their city.

My goal is not to eradicate the game. I want to alert parents and players to safety issues that need to be considered. They need to be aware of how to recognize a concussion and treat it with respect. It is not a "ding."

Every family needs to be able to recognize performance enhancing substances for their long term danger to the players' bodies. We, as a society, need to learn to play with our natural bodies; not those that are enhanced to super-human proportions.

I am certain that the NFL will continue to look at rule changes that will prevent serious injuries. It is not in their best interest financially, or publicity-wise to have seriously injured players on the field.

Since I have been quoted in the media about head injuries and have been very upfront about my own concussions, I have been sought out by a number of retired players in a variety of sports. Since I have been definitively diagnosed with several concussions, they ask me about residual problems.

Do you have migraines?

Do you get dizzy?

Do you forget where you are going or what you are talking about?

Do you have headaches and just bad days?

Each man is asking me in his own way, does he have the after effects of concussions?

Does he have brain damage?

Will he be a victim of CTE?

I answer these questions honestly. "Yes" to all the above. Right there, a bond is created. These are my friends for now and evermore. We share a fate that is being studied daily. A cure probably won't happen in time to save our brains, but our children and grandchildren may have a chance to escape the dreaded Tau protein. At the least, we suffer migraines and headaches. The good news is that the players find solace in the fact that I understand their predicament. We are alike in more ways than ever before. We are playing on the same side of the line. We are injured but pressing onward daily.

Being realistic about the prospect of continued injuries, I formed a non-profit organization to assist retired players in accessing the benefits to which they are entitled. The Gay Culverhouse Players' Outreach Program, Inc. maintains a toll free number and a website to inform players of benefit programs.

If a player needs a medical exam to quality for an NFL benefit and cannot afford it, we make it happen at no cost. We are a non-political group that is self- sufficient. We travel to players or fly players to Tampa. To insure that former players know about what we offer, we fly to the NFL cities and present at their retired players' meetings. If one group is having a golf tournament or a Super Bowl event, we attend and make certain to spread the word to the players about what we can offer them.

We ask them to find their former roommate or lineman. We look for the players that are lost to the system. We look for the homeless players. There are players living under viaducts in New Orleans, there is a player in Houston living in a FEMA trailer without electricity or water. The police picked up a player walking down the center of a major highway.

These are the men we seek for their safety and the safety of their loved ones. These men, due to CTE, can have radical personality changes that lead to violent episodes. Wives call us concerned for theirs and their children's well being. They will say, for example, that their husband has threatened to kill them with a baseball bat. We take every call seriously. We don't want harm to come to a player or his family or an innocent bystander. These former heroes of the gridiron can morph into men you do not want to know.

Is it difficult working with these men? Absolutely. They don't remember what you have told them. They may want you to help them that second, or they may curse you the next day and not want your help. I have taken calls at one in the morning. If a man is desperate, it doesn't matter what time of day or night it is. I am often times surprised by who is calling. These are men you have seen on television and who wear Super Bowl rings. Others you have never heard of and never will.

They are all in trouble.

Whether they made millions or thousands; whether they played ten years or ten months, they are in trouble. This is what I have committed myself to doing with a very capable and patient staff. This is not the stuff of glory, but of sadness.

Throughout this past year, we noticed that women are the ones who call us about their brother, son, husband, or boyfriend, so we recently added a women's program to our outreach efforts.

Women are the first to recognize the behavioral changes that signify a change in mental status. The women are the ones that make the appointments and do the follow-up paperwork that is required to obtain NFL benefits. They even set the GPS for their man to find the doctor's office for evaluations. Interestingly, one player left us after his interview confidently driving out of the parking area only to return shortly. His GPS needed to be set to return him to his home.

Eleanor Perfetto, whose husband Ralph Wentzel is a recipient of the 88 Plan's assisted living benefit, is working with me to speak with women in the NFL cities. We inform them what to look for and when and how to get help for their loved one. There is also a phone line dedicated for these women in need. We feel this program adds to our existing outreach and will be highly successful in spreading the information and helping moms and sisters, wives, and girlfriends cope with the post trauma of football.

We are creating the Lee Roy Selmon Center at the University of South Florida in honor of our first draft pick. Lee Roy is helping us design a center to meet all the aspects a retired player may encounter in his post-football life. This runs from financial management to surgery and physical therapy. Ours will be the first such center devoted to the athlete.

Training sideline personnel for Pop Warner and youth leagues as well as high school and college teams is an important component of our community outreach program. Parent education is our top priority.

A long range goal is to provide assisted living for retired players in an accommodation specially designed for their sizes and activity levels. The staff will be trained specifically to deal with the effects of CTE which has its own subset of symptoms including aggression and impulsivity.

Of course, from my perspective, the best scenario would be to make these issues obsolete. I'd love to know that my grandchildren will never suffer head injuries or broken bones, CTE, or arthritis.

I am, however, a realist. The National Football League taught me well. So I know that concussions will continue, and crushing blows will excite the fans from the youth league parents to the fans of the NFL teams. After all, what is football without the excitement of danger and super human effort?

One Republican from Texas accused me of trying to turn America's greatest game into flag football. That is not my intent. I want coaches and trainers to teach their players how to play the games as safely as they can. It will still be thrilling but perhaps when a player is knocked unconscious, he will be cared for appropriately so that he can play again in the future—so that he can have a normal old age and play football with his grandchildren. It wouldn't take that much to modify play and rules.

Rich McKay, president of the Atlanta Falcons, is co-chair of the NFL rules and competition committee. He and his committee proposed, and put into place, several rules in the past year that make the game safer to play. I daresay, no fan has complained. It is still an exciting game to watch. This year, more rules will be instituted to carry forward the league's commitment to reducing injuries.

My relationship with Richie goes back a long way, when he was about fifteen years old and had just moved with his family from California to Tampa. He was his high school's quarterback and always had a football video game in his hands. Although a bit shy, he always had a ready smile for my children.

Along with Rich, came his two sisters Michelle and Terry. They were California girls, beautiful, blond, and tan with gorgeous white teeth. They were also two of the nicest young women you would meet, both with their mother's great humor.

The eldest McKay son, Johnny, played ball at USC for his father and decided to follow the family to Tampa, where he became a starter for the Buccaneers. He was Doug Williams' favorite receiver because he knew Johnny would always be in the right spot when the ball was thrown. They were a great team.

Unfortunately, during a game in New Orleans, Doug drilled a pass to Johnny. He caught it but lost feeling in the palm of his hand from the force of the ball. From that point on, his career was jeopardized. If one is a receiver, one has to have the feel of the ball in one's hand. Johnny went on to study law and practice in California.

Corky, the family matriarch, was laid back and the coolest mom in the neighborhood. Since they lived six houses from mine, my children would ride their bikes over to visit and swim in her pool. On Halloween, Corky had Coach McKay handing out the candy. The neighborhood went wild. They were great neighbors. One would never know they were a football dynasty.

My father spent weeks convincing John to leave the Trojans and become the first coach for Tampa Bay's NFL franchise. John McKay was a legend. He had led the USC

Trojans to many championships and was well regarded in the NCAA and the NFL. He was considered a football mastermind. In retrospect one wonders what it was that convinced him to leave the glory of worship he experienced in California to become the coach of a new team.

After twenty-six straight NFL loses, McKay was defiled in the media. His star was tarnished. Johnny Carson did skits on national television about our team's inept play.

But in all fairness, in those days an expansion team was composed of players that other teams wanted to dump. There was no equity as there is today. We got the misfits. Coach McKay turned them into a team.

By the fourth year, the Bucs were one game away from the super bowl. They beat Philadelphia and went on to Dallas, where they lost in a scrappy game. It was the furthest any team had gone in the shortest amount of time. The '79 team is still revered in Tampa. To this day, there is a yearly celebration of that team. And truth be known, there is more community spirit surrounding the '79 victory than the Super Bowl win that came much later under Jon Gruden.

My father and John were best friends. Dad picked him up after a defeat, and they shared a cigar at 2:00 a.m. in the confines of One Buc Place reviewing the game. They were two great minds trying to figure out the key to making these men a team that would win. They played golf together on vacation and appreciated the strengths of one another. I'd say they loved each other like brothers.

That feeling carried over to the second generation. I have the feeling that if Dad had been awarded the LA Rams and we had moved to California, we would have sought out the McKay family and our journey would have continued much as it did. However, there probably would have been a few more wins initially, since the Rams were an established team.

The Culverhouse/McKay partnership was pre-destined in some way that is beyond my comprehension.

In 1974, we played our first game. Thirty-seven years later we, the children of the founders, are in the field again. We are following our fathers' footsteps. Rich, John, and I have professional degrees. We have worked in other fields. However, here we are in 2011, working in football. Rich is with the Atlanta Falcons, John is working in sports administration for the Trojans, and I am taking care of retired players in need. How does one explain that? I can only say, football gets in your blood and stays there forever.

I think of our fathers and wonder if they ever thought this would be their legacy. Our fathers loved football; it created a bond between them that could not be broken and grew game by game. We children formed the same bond. I believe there is a tacit understanding that runs in all football families. We understand each other without words. We know the devastating feeling of a loss at a critical time in the season. AND we know what it's like to lose a favorite player to an injury. You get a sinking feeling in the pit of your being when a player does not rise from the field. You know this man. He is part of your football family. Fans will never understand what these injuries do to us.

So to come full circle, I work with the former players through the Gay Culverhouse Players' Outreach Program, Inc., bridging the gap for the NFL from the myriad of services they offer to the actual men who need the services. I applaud the NFL for their efforts on behalf of the retired players and think they are generous in their offerings (a list follows). I am fortunate to be able to work with them to get this knowledge into the hands of the men who need it. Every time we successfully place a player in a program, we celebrate. Every time a knee is successfully replaced, we are thrilled. The NFL is trying to do the right thing.

With Rich McKay making the game safer and John working with college coaches and players, I feel that the McKay-Culverhouse partnership begun by our fathers has continued into the next generation. We shall make a difference each in our own way for the betterment of the game at all levels.

NFL PLAYER BENEFITS

"88 Plan" Dementia Benefits

Named for Pro Football Hall of Famer and NFLPA legend John Mackey, the 88 Plan is the first program of its kind in this country. The 88 Plan provides retired players with up to $88,000 per year for medical and custodial care resulting from dementia, including Alzheimer's. Funding for dementia research is also being provided. Already well over $1 million has been distributed to suffering players and their families through this benefit.

NFL Player Care Plan

Assisted Living Benefits

Three designated Assisted Living Facilities have been selected to meet the special needs of vested former players. Negotiated discounted rates and special services are made available to former players at these leading national assisted living providers – Brookdale Senior Living, Inc., Belmont Village LP, and Silverado Senior Living, Inc.

NFL Player Joint Replacement Benefit

In October 2007, the NFL added a joint replacement benefit to its Player Care Plan. This benefit is designed to assist all vested, retired players in need of knee, hip or shoulder replacements. The benefit assists players in gaining access to a nationwide network of excellent healthcare facilities and coordinated care. The plan also reimburses eligible players for up to the $5,250 towards the cost of joint replacement surgery.

Tripled Widow and Surviving Children Benefits

For a player who dies before his retirement benefits commence, the minimum death benefit paid to his widow and any surviving minor children has been tripled. Minimum monthly death benefits now range from $3,600 to $9,000.

Disability Benefits

(under the Bert Bell/Pete Rozelle NFL Player Retirement Plan and the NFL Player Supplemental Disability Plan)

"Re-opener" for Retirees Who Took Pension Early

Players who took their NFL pension early, and therefore made themselves ineligible to apply for and receive disability benefits, were offered a new one-time opportunity to apply for total and permanent disability benefits. These players were able to establish their disability through either a medical examination or by a total and permanent disability determination from Social Security.

Addition of a Medical Director for Initial Claims

The Bell/Rozelle Retirement Plan has retained a Medical Director to consult and assist with the Disability Initial Claims Committee and the Retirement Board. This should reduce the number of "deemed denials" and expedite the processing of appeals.

Establishment of Physician Panels for More Coordinated Care

Teams of physicians are being established in Arizona, California, Florida and Texas (where there is the highest concentration of retired players) in order to better coordinate retired player medical care. These physician panels, consisting of experts in orthopedic and other pertinent fields, will create a one-stop shop for players requiring comprehensive services. Physician panels in other major metropolitan areas will be added in the future.

Toll-Free Telephone Intake for Easier Application

An additional toll-free number has been established at the Plan Office to allow applicants to speak with an intake specialist to help them prepare their disability application and advise them on the process. The application processing review period begins only after the completed, signed application is received.

E-Ballot Appeals Voting for Retirement Board

Whenever possible, the Retirement Board now attempts to decide appeals via e-ballots, so that decisions do not necessarily have to wait until the next scheduled Retirement Board meeting.

Reduced Continuation Reviews on T&P Benefits

Under most circumstances, players receiving T&P benefits now only have to go through a continuation review every five years (as opposed to the previous three).

Refining the Standard for T&P Designations

The Reed Group, in conjunction with the NFL and NFLPA, is working to further refine the standards used to determine Total & Permanent disability decisions.

Retroactive Payments

For applications received on or after April 1, 2008, an award of a Total & Permanent Disability benefit under the Plan is paid retroactive to the first day of the month that is two months prior to the date of application.

Research Programs

Expanded Cardiovascular Health Screenings

Dr. Archie Roberts and Dr. Jeffrey Boone conduct 500 extensive cardiovascular health screenings of players a year. These two doctors, funded by the NFL Player Care Foundation, are working with medical centers throughout the country to conduct these cardiovascular screenings without cost in order to gather important medical information for research. Players found to be in need of cardiovascular care receive assistance in finding medical, nutritional and other treatment. Obesity screening and education are also provided.

Prostate Cancer Screenings

In conjunction with the American Urological Association, the NFL Player Care Foundation has funded a comprehensive program for prostate cancer screenings to further research and education in this area.

Notice to Active Players and Vested Former Players

IMPORTANT CHANGES AND IMPROVEMENTS IN DISABILITY BENEFITS

Increased "Inactive" T&P Benefits: Beginning April 1, 2008, the minimum Inactive total and permanent ("T&P") disability benefit will, in general, be increased to $40,000 per year ($3,333 per month). In general, benefits are reduced by 25% for players who elect an Early Payment Benefit. In a few cases, this reduction may be less. This amount applies to players who receive Inactive T&P benefits, now or in the future, and for players who converted from Inactive T&P benefits to retirement benefits.

T&P Disability Payment Starting Date: Beginning with applications for T&P benefits that are received on or after April 1, 2008 which are approved, T&P disability payments will begin as of the first day of the month that is two months prior to the date the application is received. For example, if an application received April 15, 2008 is later approved, benefits will be paid effective February 1, 2008.

If the DICC or the Retirement Board finds that an application was delayed because of mental incapacity, it may award retroactive benefits for up to 36 months, but only if and to the extent that the mental incapacity caused the delay.

No other retroactive T&P benefits will be paid for applications received after March 31, 2008. If you believe you may qualify for more than two months of retroactive benefits under the present rules, you should apply for T&P benefits no later than March 31, 2008.

For example, if you have not yet elected to receive retirement benefits and believe that you can demonstrate that you became unable to work prior to February 2008, or that Social Security found you unable to work prior to February 2008, you should apply for T&P benefits no later than March 31, 2008.

Extended Period to Apply for Line-of-Duty Disability Benefits: Beginning with applications received on or after April 1, 2008, the time to apply for LOD benefits will be extended. The new time to apply will be the greater of four years or the number of years equal to your number of Credited Seasons after you cease to be an active player. For example, a player with 10 Credited Seasons will be able to apply for LOD benefits at any time up to 10 years after he ceases to be an active player.

Recognition of Social Security Disability: Any player who is eligible for T&P benefits and who demonstrates that he is receiving Social Security disability benefits because he is unable to work will be deemed to satisfy the criteria of being totally and permanently disabled. For applications received prior to May 1, 2008, T&P benefits will be paid retroactively to the later of (1) April 1, 2007 or (2) the date Social Security has determined to be the date of disability. The appropriate category of T&P benefit – Active Football, Active Non-football, Football Degenerative, or Inactive – will be made in accordance with the terms of the Plan

Spine Treatment Program

Added to the Player Care Plan in June 2009, the NFL spine treatment program makes available spine specialists at five hospitals to evaluate and treat spine-related conditions among retired players. The program will assist players with coordinated care at excellent healthcare facilities nationwide. Each hospital provides an orthopedic spine surgeon who serves as a program director and coordinates the services of a team of health care professionals in the evaluation and, if warranted, treatment of eligible former players. The team includes a neurosurgeon and a physiatrist. Eligible players who cannot afford treatment may apply to the NFL Player Care Foundation for a grant to cover some or all of the costs of treatment.

Prescription Drug Discount Card for Retirees

Thousands of retired players have already received their new Prescription Drug Discount Card. This card, provided to players and their families' free-of-charge, is accepted at more than 57,000 pharmacies nationwide and can be used for discounts on all prescription medications.

Bibliography

Batista, Judy, "Steelers Ben Roethlisberger Says He Has Recovered from Concussion," *New York Times*, AP, January 6, 2009.

Bloomberg.com., March 17, 2008, "Athletes Don't Benefit from Human Growth Hormone, Study Finds," *Stanford University Study published in the Annals of Internal Medicine*. March 17, 2008.

Bruntz, Michael, "Football Players Feel the Need to Gain Weight," *Daily Nebraskan*. July 13, 2008.

Chaney, Mathew L., "Spiral of Denial," Four Walls, 2009.

Dulac, Gerry, "Big Ben Has Spinal Cord Concussion," *Pittsburgh Post Gazette*. January 12, 2009.

Eisenberg, John, "For McCrary, Football Took a Painful Toll." *Baltimore Sun,* May 2, 2007, nflretirees.blogspot.com/2007/05/for-mccrary-football-took-painful-toll.html, retrieved 3-27-10.

Ehrnberg, Christer and Rosen, Thord, "Physiological and Pharmacological Basis for the Ergogenic Effects of Growth Hormone in Elite Sports," *Asian Journal of Andrology*, Vol.10, issue 3, p. 373-383. Published online April 21, 2008.

Fryer, Alex, "Final Hours of DuBose's Life Recounted-Questions Linger over Death after Confrontation with Police," *The Seattle Times*. July 30, 1999.

Fryer, Alex, "Dubose Shooting Ruled Justified by San Diego District Attorney," *The Seattle Times*. November 1, 1999.

Grant, Alan, "Roughstuff: John Lynch Likes Friend's Life Confrontation, But He Will Never Understand the One That Took His Best Friend's Life," *Chicago-Sun Times*. November 19, 2000.

Gross, Daniel, "Blue Collar Workers," *New York Times*. January 21, 2007).

Froelich, Paula with Hoffmann, Bill and Steindler, Corynne, "Dan Clark's Sex Life" *New York Post*. January 1, 2009.

Hargrove, Thomas, "Heavy NFL Players Twice as Likely to Die before Age 50," Scripps Howard News Service. January 31, 2006.

Henderson, Joe, "Pro Football Bigger, Faster, and Some Say, More Dangerous," *Tampa Tribune*. January 31, 2009.

Hickson, R.C., Ball, K.l., Falduto, M.T., "Adverse Effects of Anabolic Steroids," *Medical Toxicology Adverse Drug Experiences*. 1989. July-August; 4(4): 254-71. "

Gray, Timothy, *Physics of Football,*. New York: Harper Collins. 2005.

Leiber, Jill, "Getting Physical and Chemical," *Sports Illustrated*. May 13, 1985.

Livingston, Seth, "Fight against Steroids Gaining Muscle in High School Athletics," *USA Today*. March 5, 2008.

Nelson, Glen,"Puzzling End to Life of Intensity," *The Seattle Times*. August 8, 1999.

O'Keeffe, Michael, "Once the NFL's 'Dirtiest', Conrad Dobler Tries to Piece Life Together After Football Ravaged His Health," *New York Daily News.com* January 17, 2010, nydailynews.com/ sports/ football/ 2010/01/16/2010-01-16/-conrad-dobler-trys.

Omalu, M.D. Bennet, *Play Hard, Die Young*, Lodi, CA. Neo-Forenxis Books. 2008.

Prine, Carl, "Bloody Sundays," *Pittsburgh Tribune Review*. January 9, 2005.

Peters, Jason, *Hero of the Underground,* Peters, Jason with O'Neill, Tony, St. Martin's Press, NY, NY. 2008.

Schwarz, Alan, "Silence on Concussions Raises Risks of Injuries." *New York Times,* September 15, 2007.

Schwarz, Alan, "Dark Days Follow Hard-Hitting Career in the N.F.L.," *New York Times,* February 7, 2007.

Schwarz, Alan, "Player Silence on Concussions May Block N.F.L. Guidelines," *New York Times,* June 20, 2007.

Shapiro, Leonard, "After Football, a Tragic Freefall," *The Washington Post.* November 24, 2004. p. D 01.

Silver, Marc D. MD., *The American Academy of Orthopaedic Surgeons,* vol. 9, No. 1, January/February, 2001, 61-70.

Trenton, Adam J.; Currier, Glen N., "Behavioral Manifestations of Anabolic Steroid Us," *CNS Drugs.* 2005. 19(7): 571-595.

Zinser, Lynn., "Florida State Penalized in Academic Fraud Case," *New York Times.* March 7, 2008.

AEJMC Archives, "Sports Illustrated, War on Drugs, Agenda Building and Political Timing," 1996, list.msu.edu/cgi- bin/ wa?A2=ind 9612C&L=aejmc&P=5756, en.wikiedia.org/wiki/Steve_Courson.

Wikipedia, "Steroid Use in American Football."

"Mike Webster 1952-2002," www. sportsencyclopedia.com/memorial/pit/webster.

cogscilibrarian.blogspot.com/2008/09/concussion-study-among-athletes.html, "Concussion Study among Athletes," September 28, 2008.

www.usatoday.com/sports/football/nfl/2007-06-18-concussions-cover_N.html.

Increased Heart Risks Seen for Retired NFL Players., Washingtonpost.com/nflretirees.blogspot.com/2008/04/increased-heart-risk-seen-for-retired.html, retrieved 3-24-2010.

Posted March 3, 2008 by Retired Players, "N.F.L. and N.F.L.P.A. Announce Expanded Disability Benefits Program for Retired Players." retiredplayers.org/2008/03/03/NFL-and-NFLPA-announce-expanded-disabiltiy-benefirs-program-for-retired-players.

ESPN.com., "Under Fire at Hearing, N.F.L.P.A. Seeks Help from Congress," September 18, 2007.

"Legal Issues Relating to Football Head Injuries (Part I and II), Hearings before the Committee on the Judiciary House of Representatives, One Hundred Eleventh Congress, October 28, 2009, and January 4, 2010, Serial No, 111-82. Washington, DC. U.S. Government Printing Office. 2010, also available, judiciary.house.gov.

IN APPRECIATION

To those of you who had to listen to me gnash my teeth in anger and frustration, I thank you for keeping me sane.

For Kathryn and Lorie who kept me in pound cake for brain fuel, I thank you.

For Caroline without whom this book would never exist, I'll never be able to thank you.

For Louise who urged me on and sent me every bit of research imaginable, I thank you.

For Mitchell who carries the weight of GCPOP on his shoulders, I thank you.

For my family, may you forever be protected.

For Jarek who keeps me on the field, I thank you.

For Michael who gives me great joy, I thank you.

For Bobby who keeps me focused on what really matters, I thank you.

To Alan Schwarz: don't stop!

This book was a team effort of many smart minds, and I hope I have given them justice.

I thank you for the time you gave me in pursuit of the truth.